Radiological Anatomy for FRCR Part 1

Philip Borg • Abdul Rahman J. Alvi
Nicholas T. Skipper • Christopher S. Johns

Radiological Anatomy for FRCR Part 1

Second Edition

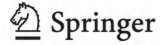

Philip Borg, MD, FRCR
Interventional Oncology Fellow
The Christie Hospital Manchester
Manchester
UK

Nicholas T. Skipper, BSc, MBBS
Radiology Registrar
Sheffield Teaching Hospitals
Sheffield
UK

Abdul Rahman J. Alvi, MBBS, MRCS
Radiology Intervention Fellow
Royal Free Hospital
London
UK

Christopher S. Johns, MBBS
Radiology Registrar
Sheffield Teaching Hospitals
Sheffield
UK

ISBN 978-3-642-41165-6   ISBN 978-3-642-41166-3   (eBook)
DOI 10.1007/978-3-642-41166-3
Springer Heidelberg New York Dordrecht London

Library of Congress Control Number: 2014933791

Printed on acid-free paper

Springer is part of Springer Science+Business Media (www.springer.com)

Foreword to the Second Edition

Both diagnostic radiology and interventional radiology are wonderful careers. Unfortunately the exam is a necessary evil. Anything that can be done to smooth the passage through to success is to be welcomed. The previous edition of this book, with its associated e-learning modules, was a run-away success, testament to the content and value of a well-constructed concept that will ease examinees through the anatomy part of FRCR. The new text and e-learning has been extensively reworked with lots of new questions, new subjects and new contributors. The authors are to be congratulated on what will again be seen as an essential resource for gliding through the FRCR.

Peter A. Gaines
Hallam University and
Sheffield Vascular Institute

Foreword to the First Edition

Sound anatomical knowledge is the bed-rock of a good radiologist. I am pleased to say that it is some while since I had to suffer the rigor of anatomical learning only then to be examined by humourless learned gentlemen of the College. The radiology consisted largely of dusted down plain radiographs, primitive CT and nuclear medicine composed of bricks rather than pixels (although that doesn't seem to have changed much).

Happily both imaging and the way that anatomy is examined have changed immeasurably. The preface deals with the change in the examination. Imaging has become more diverse and the anatomical detail is refined. This means that all students need to have an exquisite knowledge of anatomy in multiple planes using numerous imaging modalities. This book and its associated on-line modules parallel the new imaging and the way the curriculum is examined. The structure will not only give students of anatomy practice at the exam, but will also deliver an enjoyable way of learning.

Peter A. Gaines
Hallam University and
Sheffield Vascular Institute

Preface to the Second Edition

Three years after the publication of the first edition, this book remains the best seller in its category and has sold over a thousand copies worldwide. The second edition has been designed to reflect the change in format of the exam introduced in Spring 2013. It also includes two new chapters as well as a few new cases in the remainder of the chapters from the first edition.

The new exam format consists of 100 cases with a single question per case (a change from the previous 20 cases with 5 questions per case). A single mark will be answered for the correct answer, which also includes the correct side when possible. There will be no negative marking. The level of anatomical knowledge required to successfully pass the exam has not changed. From feedback we have received, the questions in this book reflect the level of difficulty found in the exam. We wish you the best of luck in your exams and your careers!

P.B.
A.R.J.A.
N.T.S.
C.S.J.

Preface to the First Edition

The new format FRCR part 1 anatomy exam was introduced in March 2010. This book has been written to allow candidates to identify the level of anatomical knowledge expected by the college and to provide a self-assessment tool providing candidates with valuable practice before the exam. The aim of this book is to supplement, not replace, established radiology anatomy textbooks and atlases.

In the exam the cases will be viewed using Osirix software on an Apple Mac mini workstation with a 19″ monitor. The current format comprises 20 cases/images, with 5 questions about each. As a candidate you have 75 min in which to complete the exam. The images are labelled 1–20 and the 5 questions are labelled (a) to (e). You will be provided with a question booklet into which you write your answers. It is imperative that your answers are legible to secure full marks.

In-depth knowledge and the ability to describe anatomy is an integral part of radiology. As in clinical practice, the college stresses the importance of labelling the correct side of the structure. For each question the RCR awards 2 marks, 1 mark is awarded for correctly naming the structure and another for describing the correct side.

We advise that you approach each image as if you were viewing these images in real life and adopt a system to interpret them thus ensuring that you have identified both the correct side and structure.

An axial section of a CT or MRI is displayed as if the body were viewed from below. In the current exam format, you are presented with a single slice of an image in the axial, sagittal or coronal plane. This sometimes may lead to ambiguity about the correct answer as you do not have the facility to scroll up and down the image to corroborate your answer. The RCR, in these instances, may allow for more than one correct answer.

The questions in this book have been arranged in a similar format to the exam and we have tried to cover all imaging modalities and included cases that are most likely to be assessed. We encourage attempting these tests under exam conditions. By working through each test, we hope that you will gain confidence in your knowledge of the key topics as well as identify areas that may require further study. No cases have been repeated but some that are similar represent the cases that we think are important and likely to feature in the exam. In some instances, more than one correct answer has been listed to allow for the difference in nomenclature sometimes encountered.

Separate chapters on paediatric imaging and anatomical variants have been included as questions on these topics have been included in the previous examination.

Where appropriate, information has been provided after the answers including useful hints on how to accurately identify structures using various landmarks and aide-memoires. There is also information for questions other than 'name the structure' that may be asked. This information should aid further revision from the recommended textbooks and atlases currently available.

Finally, we wish you the best of luck in your exams and your careers.

P.B.
A.R.J.A.

Contents

Contributors

Jane C. Belfield, MBChB, MRCP, FRCR Royal Liverpool University Hospital, Liverpool, UK

Devendranath Betarse, MBBS, MRCS, FRCR Leeds Teaching Hospitals, Leeds, England, UK

Matthew J. Bull, MBChB, FRCR University of Sheffield, Sheffield Teaching Hospitals, Sheffield, England, UK

Daniel J.A. Connolly, BSc, MRCP, FRCR University of Sheffield, Sheffield Teaching Hospitals NHS Trust, Sheffield, England, UK

Peter A. Gaines, MBChB, FRCP, FRCR Sheffield Vascular Institute, University of Sheffield, Sheffield, England, UK

David Hughes, BSc, MBChB, MRCP, FRCR Sheffield Children's Hospital, Sheffield, England, UK

Test 1

(You have 90 minutes to complete 100 questions)

P. Borg et al., *Radiological Anatomy for FRCR Part 1*,
DOI 10.1007/978-3-642-41166-3_1, © Springer-Verlag Berlin Heidelberg 2014

CT Chest

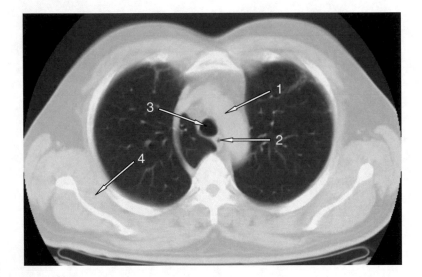

Questions	
1.	Name the structure labelled 1.
2.	Name the structure labelled 2.
3.	Name the structure labelled 3.
4.	Name the structure labelled 4.
5.	What normal variant is present in this image?

MRI Knee

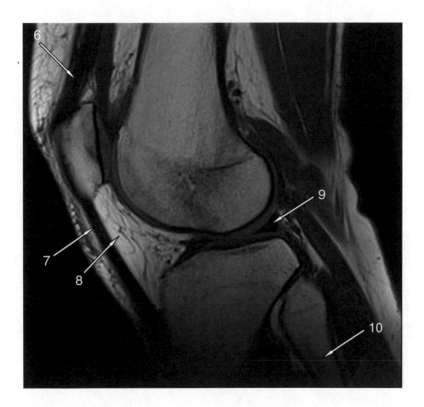

Questions	
6.	Name the structure labelled 6.
7.	Name the structure labelled 7.
8.	Name the structure labelled 8.
9.	Name the structure labelled 9.
10.	Name the structure labelled 10.

Skull Radiograph

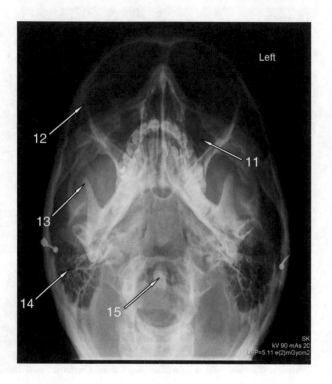

Questions	
11.	Name the structure labelled 11.
12.	Name the structure labelled 12.
13.	Name the structure labelled 13.
14.	Name the structure labelled 14.
15.	Name the structure labelled 15.

Ultrasound Abdomen

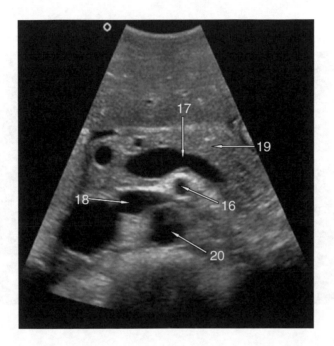

Questions	
16.	Name the structure labelled 16.
17.	Name the structure labelled 17.
18.	Name the structure labelled 18.
19.	Name the structure labelled 19.
20.	Name the structure labelled 20.

MRI Pelvis

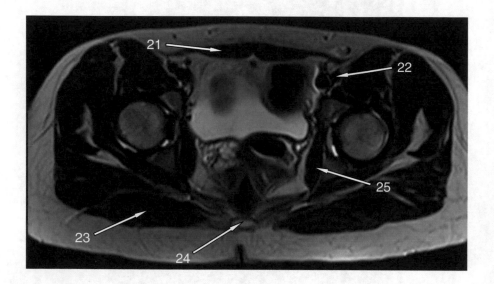

Questions	
21.	Name the structure labelled 21.
22.	Name the structure labelled 22.
23.	Name the structure labelled 23.
24.	Name the structure labelled 24.
25.	Name the structure labelled 25.

Elbow Radiograph

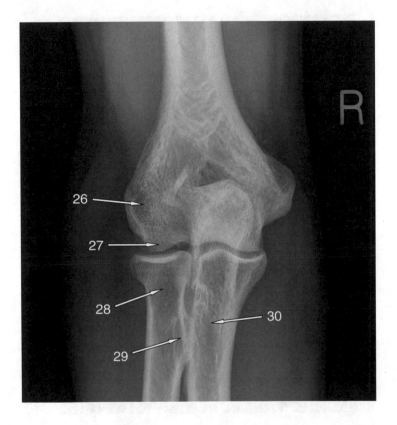

Questions	
26.	Name the structure labelled 26.
27.	Name the structure labelled 27.
28.	Name the structure labelled 28.
29.	What muscle inserts into structure 29?
30.	Name the structure labelled 30.

Hand Radiograph

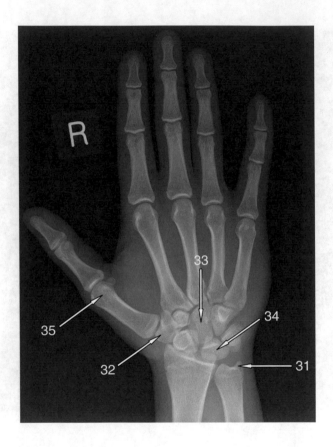

Questions	
31.	Name the structure labelled 31.
32.	Name the structure labelled 32.
33.	Name the structure labelled 33.
34.	Name the structure labelled 34.
35.	Name the structure labelled 35.

Barium Swallow

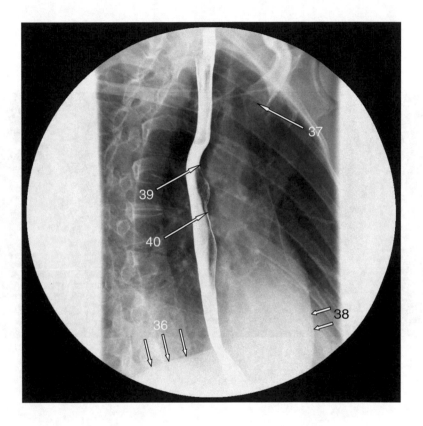

Questions	
36.	Name the structure labelled 36.
37.	Name the structure labelled 37.
38.	Name the structure labelled 38.
39.	What structure causes this impression?
40.	What structure causes this impression?

CT Chest

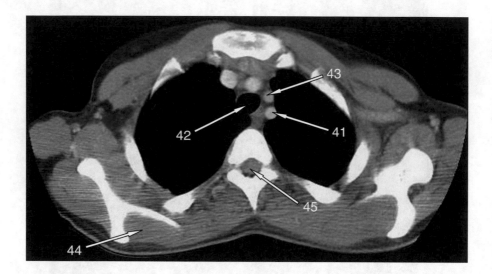

Questions	
41.	Name the structure labelled 41.
42.	Name the structure labelled 42.
43.	Name the structure labelled 43.
44.	Name the structure labelled 44.
45.	Name the structure labelled 45.

MRI Brain

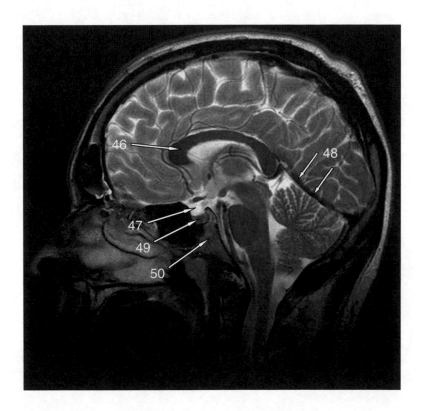

Questions	
46.	Name the structure labelled 46.
47.	Name the structure labelled 47.
48.	Name the structure labelled 48.
49.	Name the structure labelled 49.
50.	Name the structure labelled 50.

MRI Brain

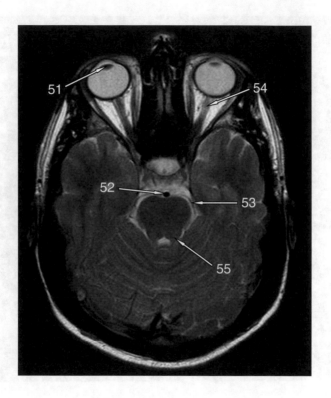

Questions	
51.	Name the structure labelled 51.
52.	Name the structure labelled 52.
53.	Name the structure labelled 53.
54.	Name the structure labelled 54.
55.	Name the structure labelled 55.

MRI Spine

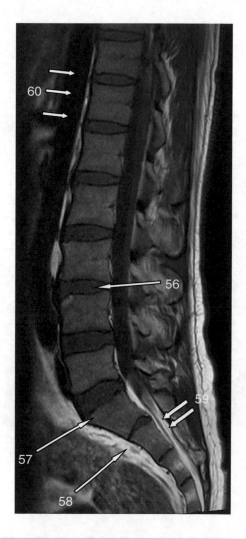

Questions	
56.	Name the structure labelled 56.
57.	Name the structure labelled 57.
58.	Name the structure labelled 58.
59.	Name the structure labelled 59.
60.	Name the structure labelled 60.

Pelvic Radiograph

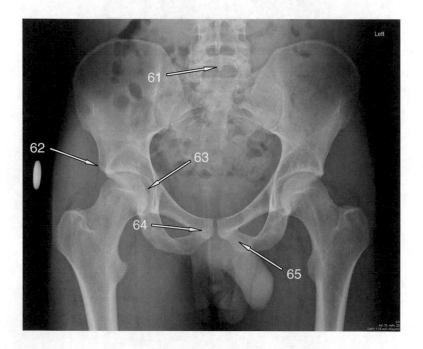

Questions	
61.	Name the structure labelled 61.
62.	Name the structure labelled 62.
63.	Name the structure labelled 63.
64.	Name the structure labelled 64.
65.	Name the structure labelled 65.

CT Abdomen

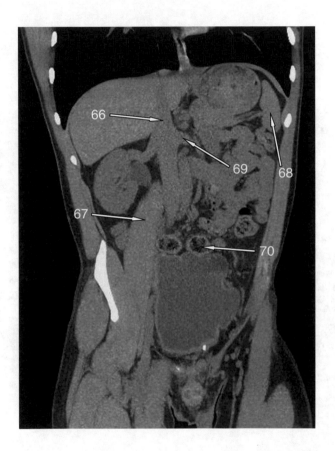

Questions	
66.	At what vertebral level does structure 66 traverse the diaphragm?
67.	Name the structure labelled 67.
68.	Name the structure labelled 68.
69.	Name the structure labelled 69.
70.	Name the structure labelled 70.

Barium Enema

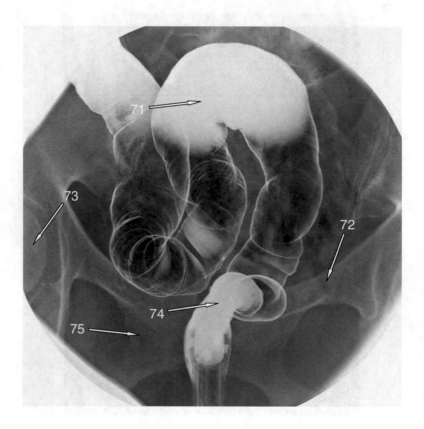

Questions	
71.	Name the structure labelled 71.
72.	Name the structure labelled 72.
73.	Name the structure labelled 73.
74.	Name the structure labelled 74.
75.	Name the structure labelled 75.

MRI Brain

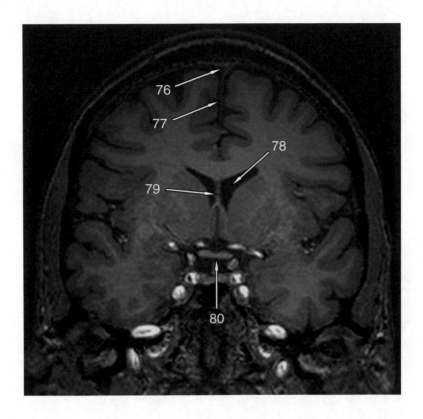

Questions	
76.	Name the structure labelled 76.
77.	Name the structure labelled 77.
78.	Name the structure labelled 78.
79.	Name the structure labelled 79.
80.	Name the structure labelled 80.

MR Angiogram

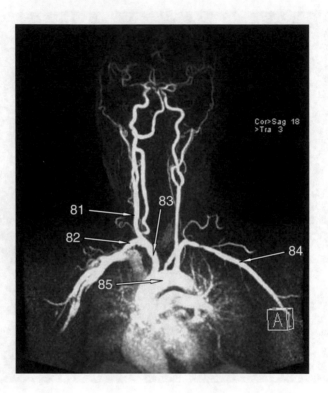

Questions	
81.	Name the structure labelled 81.
82.	Name the structure labelled 82.
83.	Name the structure labelled 83.
84.	Name the structure labelled 84.
85.	Name the structure labelled 85.

Chest Radiograph

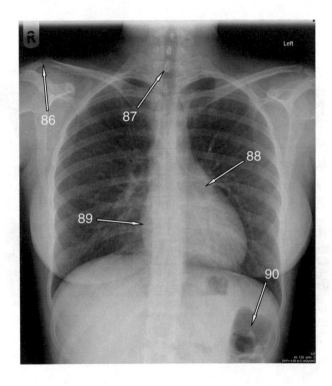

Questions	
86.	Name the structure labelled 86.
87.	Name the structure labelled 87.
88.	What part of the heart is labelled 88?
89.	What part of the heart is labelled 89?
90.	Name the structure labelled 90.

CT Pelvis

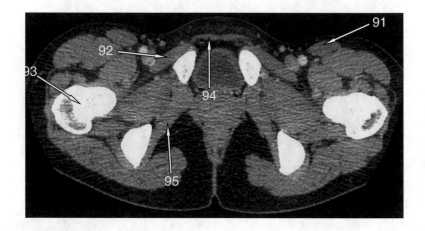

Questions	
91.	Name the structure labelled 91.
92.	Name the structure labelled 92.
93.	Name the structure labelled 93.
94.	Name the structure labelled 94.
95.	Name the structure labelled 95.

Foot Radiograph

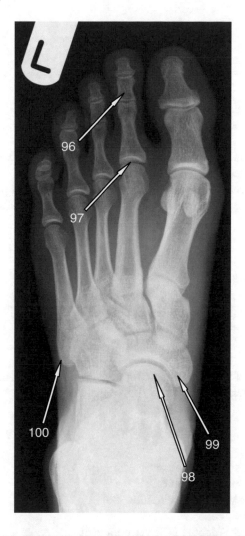

Questions	
96.	Name the structure labelled 96.
97.	Name the structure labelled 97.
98.	Name the structure labelled 98.
99.	Name the structure labelled 99.
100.	Name the structure labelled 100.

Test 1 Answers

CT Chest

1. Arch of the aorta
2. Oesophagus
3. Trachea
4. Right subscapularis muscle
5. Azygos lobe/fissure

This is the appearance of a collapsed oesophagus which is always found behind a much more easily recognised trachea.

An azygos lobe is a normal anatomical variant found in 1 % of people. It is separated from the rest of the upper lobe by two folds of parietal and two folds of visceral pleura.

MRI Knee

6. Quadriceps tendon
7. Patellar ligament
8. Hoffa's fat pad (or infrapatellar fat pad)
9. Posterior horn of lateral meniscus
10. Neck of fibula

This sagittal MRI of the knee is taken through the fibular head; therefore, the meniscus must be the lateral meniscus.

Skull Radiograph

11. Left maxillary sinus
12. Right fronto-zygomatic suture
13. Right coronoid process of mandible
14. Right mastoid air cells
15. Odontoid process (dens) of C2 vertebra (axis)

All answers have 2 marks awarded. Always label the side when possible. Even if you get the structure right, you will only be awarded one point if the side is not included in the answer.

Ultrasound Abdomen

16. Superior mesenteric artery
17. Confluence of splenic vein and superior mesenteric vein/portal vein
18. Left renal vein
19. Body of pancreas
20. Abdominal aorta

Look for the tadpole shape of the splenic vein (tail) and portal confluence (head). The pancreas is located anteriorly to the 'tadpole'.

To distinguish the aorta from the IVC: the aorta lies to the left of the IVC, is smaller in diameter and is surrounded by a concentric echo-bright area which represents peri-arterial fat.

MRI Pelvis

21. Right rectus abdominis muscle
22. Left external iliac artery
23. Right gluteus maximus muscle
24. Coccyx
25. Left obturator internus muscle

When presented with an MRI case, firstly it is important to identify the sequence. A useful hint is to remember that fluid is bright on T2-weighted images and fat is bright on T1-weighted images.

Elbow Radiograph

26. Right lateral epicondyle of humerus
27. Right capitellum of humerus
28. Right neck of radius
29. Right biceps brachii muscle
30. Right shaft of ulna

Hand Radiograph

31. Right styloid process of ulna
32. Right trapezium
33. Right capitate
34. Right lunate
35. Right head of thumb metacarpal

Phalanges and metacarpals should be named (not numbered) according to the corresponding digit, e.g. thumb not 1st metacarpal.

Barium Swallow

36. Right hemidiaphragm
37. Left medial head of clavicle
38. Anterior border of heart (right ventricle)
39. Arch of aorta
40. Left main bronchus

This barium swallow image is taken in the right anterior oblique position. Three major impressions in the oesophagus are seen anteriorly. These are made by the aortic arch, the left main bronchus and the left atrium from above down.

CT Chest

41. Left subclavian artery
42. Trachea
43. Left common carotid artery
44. Right supraspinatus muscle
45. Spinal canal (spinal cord)

The supraspinatus muscle is superior to the spine of the scapula and therefore medial to it on axial section.

MRI Brain

46. Genu of corpus callosum
47. Suprasellar cistern
48. Straight sinus
49. Pituitary gland
50. Clivus

The visible subarachnoid cisterns on a sagittal MRI of the brain include the supra-sellar cistern, interpeduncular cistern, pontine cistern, cisterna magna and quadri-geminal cistern.

MRI Brain

51. Lens of right eye
52. Basilar artery
53. Left posterior cerebral artery
54. Left optic nerve
55. Left superior cerebellar peduncle

Vessels in MR are represented as signal void (low signal) because of flow artefact. This slice is through the superior pons; structure 55 is therefore the superior cerebellar peduncle bridging between the pons and cerebellum. The superior and inferior colliculi of the quadrigeminal plate are found higher than this, at the level of the midbrain and do not bridge across to the cerebellum.

MRI Spine

56. L3/L4 intervertebral disc
57. Sacral promontory
58. Presacral space
59. Filum terminale
60. Abdominal aorta

Remember to name the different parts of the aorta (it may seem obvious but you will lose marks unnecessarily).

Pelvic Radiograph

61. Spinous process L5 vertebra
62. Right anterior inferior iliac spine
63. Right fovea capitis of femur
64. Right body of pubic bone
65. Left inferior ramus of pubic bone

CT Abdomen

66. T8
67. Right psoas major muscle
68. Spleen
69. Left renal vein
70. Small intestine (loops of)

The IVC traverses the diaphragm at T8. The levels at which important structures traverse the diaphragm can be remembered as follows: vena cava (8 letters, T8), oesophagus (10 letters, T10) and aortic hiatus (12 letters, T12).

Barium Enema

71. Sigmoid colon
72. Left superior ramus of pubis
73. Right head of femur
74. Rectum
75. Right body of pubic bone

MRI Brain

76. Superior sagittal sinus
77. Falx cerebri
78. Left lateral ventricle
79. Septum pellucidum
80. Optic chiasm

MR Angiogram

81. Right common carotid artery
82. Right subclavian artery
83. Brachiocephalic trunk
84. Left subclavian artery
85. Arch of the aorta

This is a MIP (maximum intensity projection) angiogram of the aorta and neck vessels. The cube in the bottom right-hand corner identifies the plane in which the reformatted image is being viewed (*A* for anterior, *L* for left, *P* for posterior, etc.).

Chest Radiograph

86. Right acromioclavicular joint
87. Spinous process T1 vertebra
88. Left atrium (left atrial appendage)
89. Right atrium
90. Gas in colon/splenic flexure

This is gas in the colon; the gastric air bubble is seen superiorly.

CT Pelvis

91. Left sartorius muscle
92. Right pectineus muscle
93. Right femur (right neck of femur)
94. Right rectus abdominis muscle
95. Right obturator internus muscle

Foot Radiograph

96. Left middle phalanx 2nd toe
97. Left 2nd metatarsophalangeal joint
98. Left talus (head of talus)
99. Left navicular bone
100. Left styloid process 5th metatarsal

Test 2

(You have 90 minutes to complete 100 questions)

2

P. Borg et al., *Radiological Anatomy for FRCR Part 1*,
DOI 10.1007/978-3-642-41166-3_2, © Springer-Verlag Berlin Heidelberg 2014

CT C-Spine

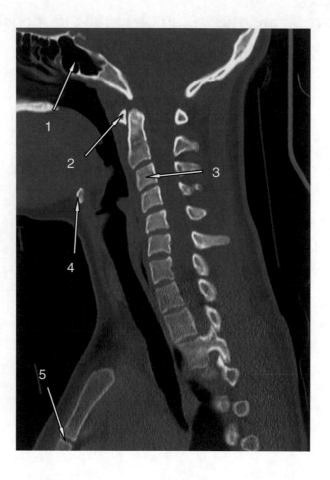

Questions	
1.	Name the structure labelled 1.
2.	Name the structure labelled 2.
3.	Name the structure labelled 3.
4.	Name the structure labelled 4.
5.	Name the structure labelled 5.

Wrist Radiograph

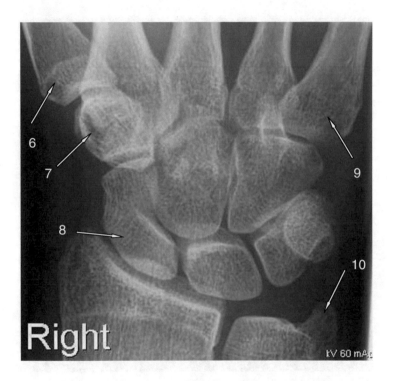

Questions	
6.	Name the structure labelled 6.
7.	Name the structure labelled 7.
8.	Name the structure labelled 8.
9.	Name the structure labelled 9.
10.	Name the structure labelled 10.

MRI Pelvis

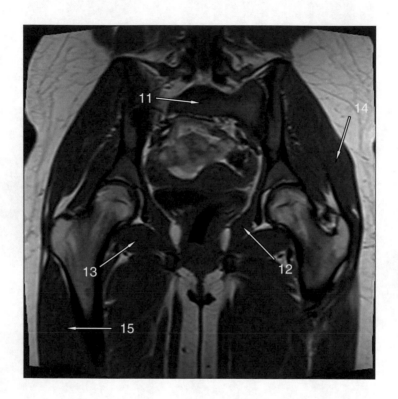

Questions	
11.	Name the structure labelled 11.
12.	Name the structure labelled 12.
13.	Name the structure labelled 13.
14.	Name the structure labelled 14.
15.	Name the structure labelled 15.

Ultrasound Pelvis

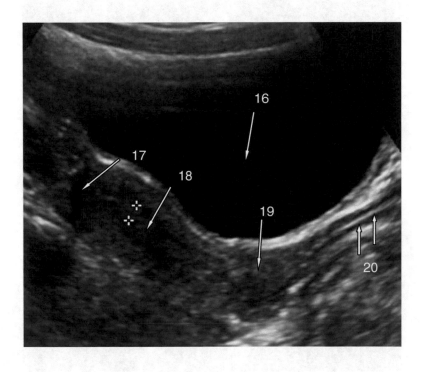

Questions	
16.	Name the structure labelled 16.
17.	Name the structure labelled 17.
18.	Name the structure labelled 18.
19.	Name the structure labelled 19.
20.	Name the structure labelled 20.

MRCP

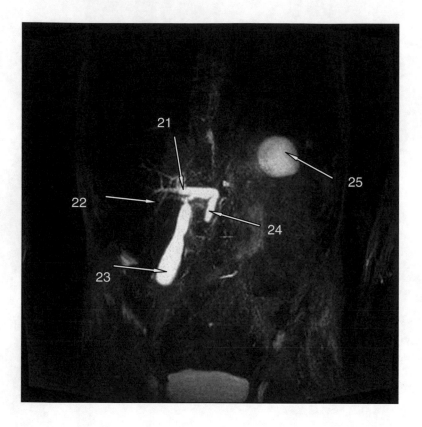

Questions	
21.	Name the structure labelled 21.
22.	Name the structure labelled 22.
23.	Name the structure labelled 23.
24.	Name the structure labelled 24.
25.	Name the structure labelled 25.

MRI Ankle

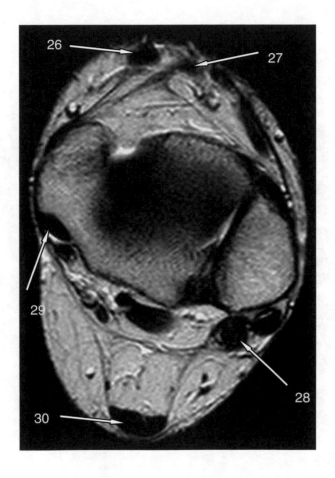

Questions	
26.	Name the structure labelled 26.
27.	Name the structure labelled 27.
28.	Name the structure labelled 28.
29.	Name the structure labelled 29.
30.	Name the structure labelled 30.

Barium Enema

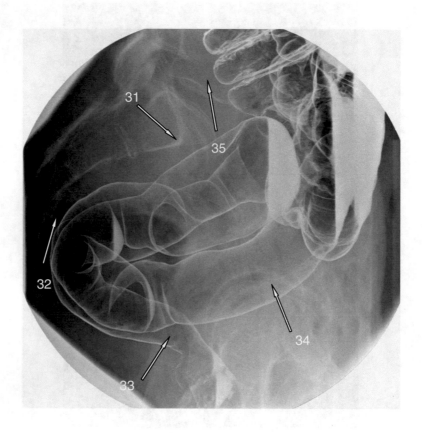

Questions	
31.	Name the structure labelled 31.
32.	Name the structure labelled 32.
33.	Name the structure labelled 33.
34.	Name the structure labelled 34.
35.	Name the structure labelled 35.

MRI Shoulder

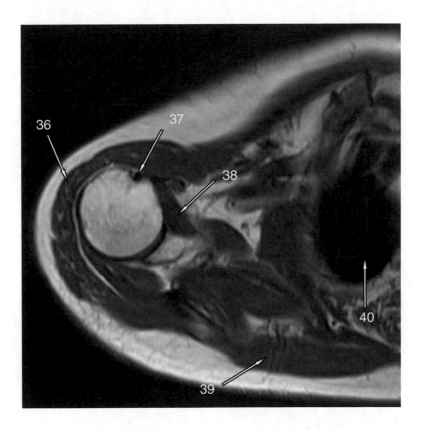

Questions	
36.	Name the structure labelled 36.
37.	Name the structure labelled 37.
38.	Name the structure labelled 38.
39.	Name the structure labelled 39.
40.	Name the structure labelled 40.

MRI Brain

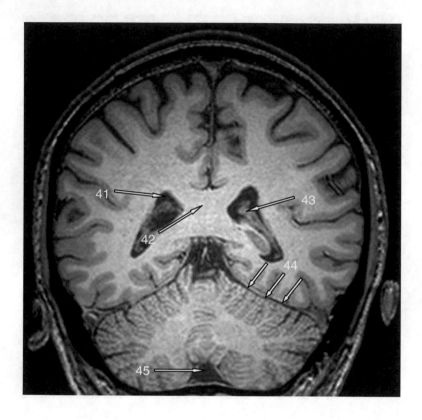

Questions	
41.	Name the structure labelled 41.
42.	Name the structure labelled 42.
43.	Name the structure labelled 43.
44.	Name the structure labelled 44.
45.	Name the structure labelled 45.

Chest Radiograph

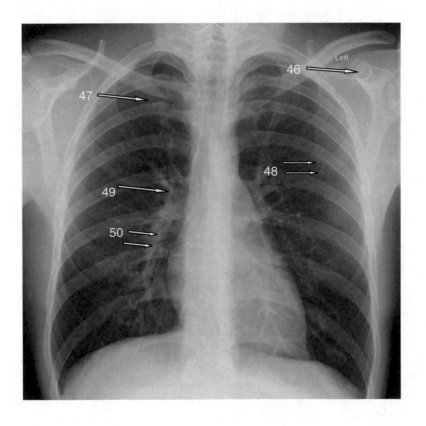

Questions	
46.	Name the structure labelled 46.
47.	Name the structure labelled 47.
48.	Name the structure labelled 48.
49.	Name the structure labelled 49.
50.	Name the structure labelled 50.

Cardiac CT

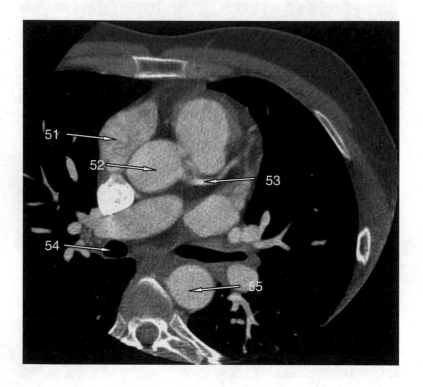

Questions	
51.	Name the structure labelled 51.
52.	Name the structure labelled 52.
53.	Name the structure labelled 53.
54.	Name the structure labelled 54.
55.	Name the structure labelled 55.

MRI Knee

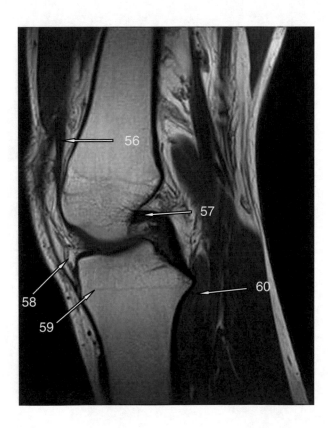

Questions	
56.	Name the structure labelled 56.
57.	Name the structure labelled 57.
58.	Name the structure labelled 58.
59.	Name the structure labelled 59.
60.	Name the structure labelled 60.

MR Angiogram

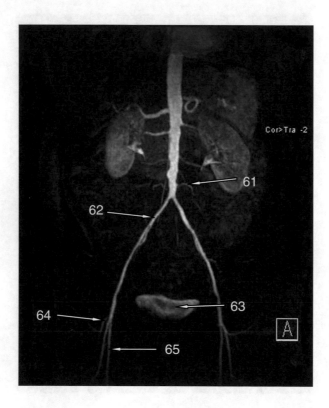

Questions	
61.	Name the structure labelled 61.
62.	Name the structure labelled 62.
63.	Name the structure labelled 63.
64.	Name the structure labelled 64.
65.	Name the structure labelled 65.

MRI Brain

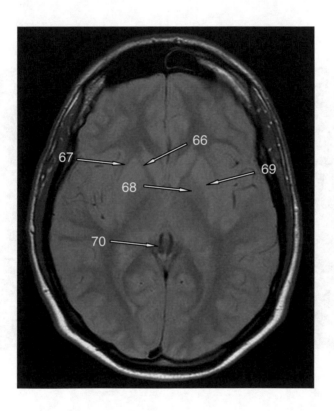

Questions	
66.	Name the structure labelled 66.
67.	Name the structure labelled 67.
68.	Name the structure labelled 68.
69.	Name the structure labelled 69.
70.	Name the structure labelled 70.

CT Foot

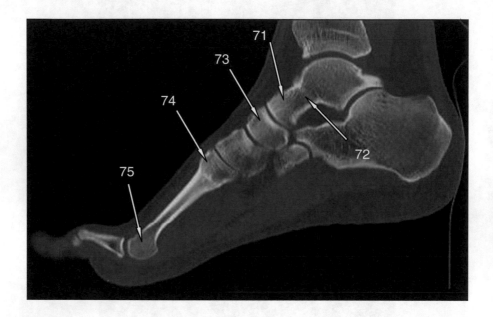

Questions	
71.	Name the structure labelled 71.
72.	Name the structure labelled 72.
73.	Name the structure labelled 73.
74.	Name the structure labelled 74.
75.	Name the structure labelled 75.

CT Abdomen

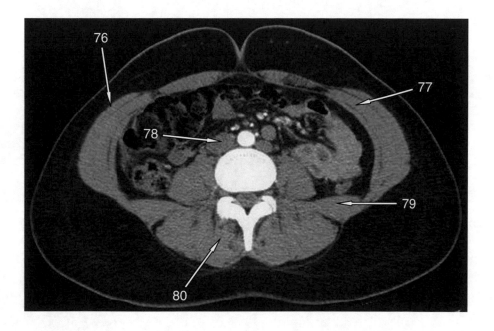

Questions	
76.	Name the structure labelled 76.
77.	Name the structure labelled 77.
78.	Name the structure labelled 78.
79.	Name the structure labelled 79.
80.	Name the structure labelled 80.

CT Chest

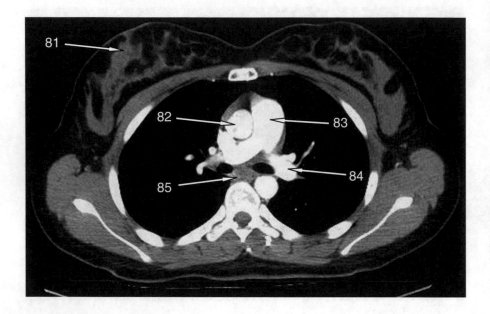

Questions	
81.	Name the structure labelled 81.
82.	Name the structure labelled 82.
83.	Name the structure labelled 83.
84.	Name the structure labelled 84.
85.	Name the structure labelled 85.

MRI Brain

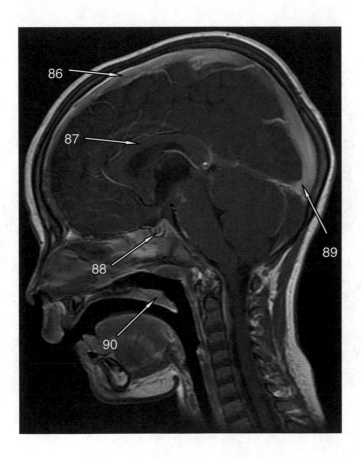

Questions	
86.	Name the structure labelled 86.
87.	Name the structure labelled 87.
88.	Name the structure labelled 88.
89.	Name the structure labelled 89.
90.	Name the structure labelled 90.

Urethrogram

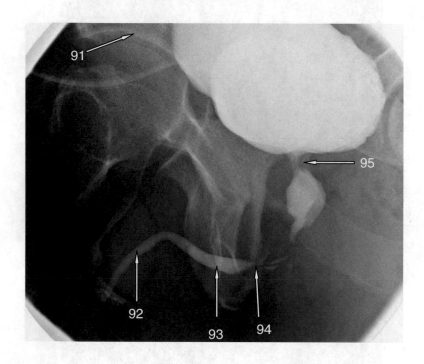

91.	Name the structure labelled 91.
92.	Name the structure labelled 92.
93.	Name the structure labelled 93.
94.	Name the structure labelled 94.
95.	Name the structure labelled 95.

MRI Knee

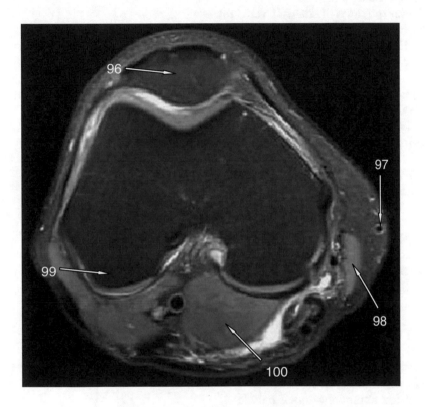

Test 2 Answers

CT C-Spine

1. Sphenoid sinus
2. Anterior arch of atlas (C1 vertebra)
3. Body of C3 vertebra
4. Hyoid bone (body of)
5. Manubrio-sternal joint

When trying to identify the vertebral level on a lateral c-spine, the odontoid process (or odontoid peg or dens) of the C2 vertebra is a useful landmark.

The manubrio-sternal joint or angle of Louis is at the approximate level of the beginning and end of the aortic arch and the bifurcation of the trachea.

Wrist Radiograph

6. Base of right thumb metacarpal
7. Right trapezium
8. Right scaphoid
9. Base of right little finger metacarpal
10. Styloid process of right ulna

MRI Pelvis

11. Sacrum/sacral promontory
12. Left obturator internus muscle
13. Right obturator externus muscle
14. Left gluteus medius muscle
15. Right vastus lateralis muscle

Ultrasound Pelvis

16. Urinary bladder
17. Myometrium
18. Endometrium
19. Cervix
20. Vagina

MRCP

21. Common hepatic duct
22. Right hepatic duct
23. Gallbladder (fundus of)
24. Common bile duct
25. Fluid in fundus of stomach

Tips: MRCP uses heavily T2-weighted sequences to utilise the properties of bile. It is a relatively quick investigation, involves no radiation and is noninvasive (compare with ERCP). Look for anatomical variations including accessory hepatic ducts, pancreas divisum and annular pancreas. The pancreatic duct should be clearly seen on MRCP.

MRI Ankle

26. Tibialis anterior tendon (left)
27. Extensor hallucis longus tendon (left)
28. Peroneus brevis tendon (left)
29. Tibialis posterior tendon (left)
30. Achilles' tendon (left)

There is no marker on the case but you can work out that it is the left lower limb (fibula on the lateral aspect).

Remember the acronym *Tom Dick Harry* (*Tibialis* posterior, flexor *Digitorum* longus, flexor *Hallucis* longus) for the tendons posterior to the medial malleolus.

For the anterior tendons *Tom Harry Dick* (*Tibialis* anterior, extensor *Hallucis* longus, extensor *Digitorum* longus).

Barium Enema

31. Sacral promontory
32. Presacral/postrectal space
33. Rectum
34. Sigmoid colon
35. L5 vertebral body

The presacral (or postrectal) space is clinically very important to determine tumour invasion and leaks following bowel anastomosis breakdown. The measurement between the anterior sacrum at the S4 level and the posterior wall of the rectum should not measure more than 4 mm.

MRI Shoulder

36. Right deltoid muscle
37. Right biceps brachii tendon (long head, in bicipital groove)
38. Right subscapularis (muscle/tendon)
39. Right infraspinatus muscle
40. Lung (apex right lung)

This is an axial T1-weighted MR shoulder.

MRI Brain

41. Right trigone of lateral ventricle
42. Splenium of corpus callosum
43. Choroid plexus (within the left lateral ventricle)
44. Tentorium cerebelli
45. Cisterna magna (cerebellomedullary cistern)

The choroid plexus is found in the lateral and third ventricles. It is responsible for CSF production.

Chest Radiograph

46. Left coracoid process
47. Right 1st rib (anterior)
48. Medial border of left scapula
49. Right hilar point
50. Interlobar artery (right lower lobe artery)

The hilar points are the angles formed by the descending upper lobe veins, as they cross behind the lower lobe arteries.

Cardiac CT

51. Right atrium
52. Aortic root
53. Left main stem coronary artery
54. Right bronchus intermedius
55. Descending thoracic aorta

The left coronary artery arises from the left posterior aortic sinus. It then divides into left anterior descending and circumflex branches. The right coronary artery arises from the anterior aortic sinus, runs in the atrioventricular groove and anastamoses with the circumflex branch of the left coronary artery.

MRI Knee

56. Quadriceps tendon
57. Posterior cruciate ligament
58. Hoffa's (infrapatellar) fat pad
59. Tibia (proximal physis)
60. Popliteus muscle

Anterior and posterior cruciate ligaments are named according to their tibial origins.
  Remember *AL, PM*: *A*nterior cruciate goes *L*ateral and *P*osterior cruciate goes *M*edial.

MR Angiogram

61. Left lumbar artery
62. Right common iliac artery
63. Urinary bladder
64. Right lateral circumflex femoral artery
65. Right superficial femoral artery

The bladder fills up with contrast in many investigations including this MRA. Always label as the 'urinary bladder'.
  The lateral circumflex femoral artery delineates the border between external iliac and femoral artery.
  Remember that the superficial femoral lies medial to the profunda femoris artery.

MRI Brain

66. Anterior limb of right internal capsule
67. Right external capsule
68. Left globus pallidus
69. Left putamen
70. Right internal cerebral vein

The globus pallidus (medial) and the putamen (lateral) make up the lentiform nucleus. The external capsule is found lateral to the lentiform nucleus.
  The internal cerebral veins are found in the quadrigeminal cistern.

CT Foot

71. Head of talus
72. Neck of talus
73. Navicular bone
74. Base of first metatarsal
75. Head of first metatarsal

CT Abdomen

76. Right external oblique muscle
77. Left internal oblique muscle
78. Inferior vena cava
79. Left quadratus lumborum muscle
80. Right erector spinae muscles

This axial CT is taken in the arterial phase of contrast enhancement. Notice how the aorta and other arteries are enhancing. Determining the phase of a CT examination is important when identifying vascular structures and pathology.

CT Chest

81. Right breast tissue
82. Ascending aorta
83. Pulmonary trunk
84. Left main pulmonary artery
85. Oesophagus

This axial CT chest (CTPA) is taken in the arterial phase. There is an apparent discontinuation between the pulmonary trunk and the left pulmonary artery because of the orientation of the slice.

Remember the oesophagus is always found behind the trachea and here behind the carina.

MRI Brain

86. Superior sagittal sinus
87. Body of corpus callosum
88. Pituitary gland
89. Torcula herophili (confluence of venous sinuses)
90. Soft palate

Urethrogram

91. Right acetabulum
92. Penile urethra
93. Bulbous urethra
94. External sphincter (sphincter urethrae)
95. Neck of bladder

This is a urethrogram, very simple to identify the anatomy if you are familiar with the procedure. Try to observe a urethrogram at least once before the exam.

MRI Knee

  96. Patella
  97. Great saphenous vein
  98. Sartorius muscle
  99. Lateral condyle of femur
100. Medial head of gastrocnemius

Identifying medial and lateral on an axial knee may be a bit tricky. Try to identify the great saphenous vein – a superficial vessel on the medial aspect in a thicker layer of superficial fat than the lateral side of the knee.

    If the menisci are visible on an axial section, the medial meniscus can be identified as the larger of the two.

Test 3

3

(You have 90 minutes to complete 100 questions)

P. Borg et al., *Radiological Anatomy for FRCR Part 1*,
DOI 10.1007/978-3-642-41166-3_3, © Springer-Verlag Berlin Heidelberg 2014

MRI Head

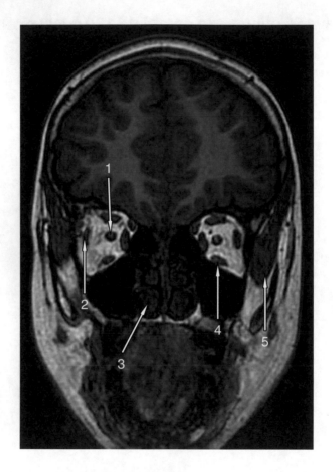

Questions	
1.	Name the structure labelled 1.
2.	What nerve supplies the structure labelled 2?
3.	Name the structure labelled 3.
4.	Name the structure labelled 4.
5.	Name the structure labelled 5.

Barium Enema

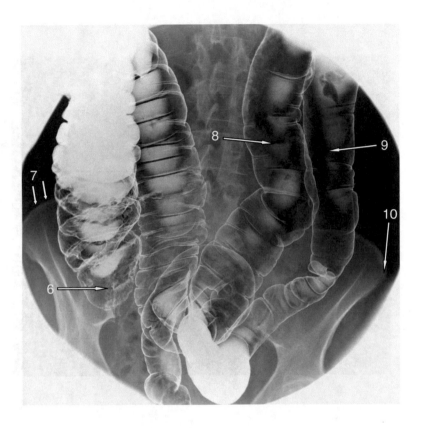

Questions	
6.	Name the structure labelled 6.
7.	Name the structure labelled 7.
8.	Name the structure labelled 8.
9.	Name the structure labelled 9.
10.	Name the structure labelled 10.

Elbow Radiograph

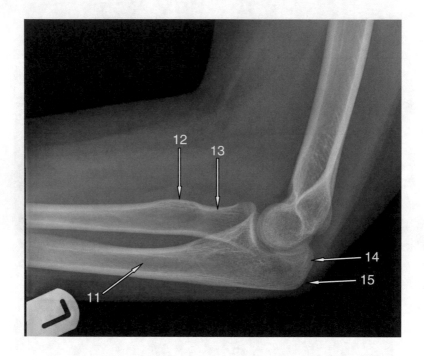

Questions	
11.	Name the structure labelled 11.
12.	Name the structure labelled 12.
13.	Name the structure labelled 13.
14.	Name the structure labelled 14.
15.	What muscle inserts into 15?

CT Chest

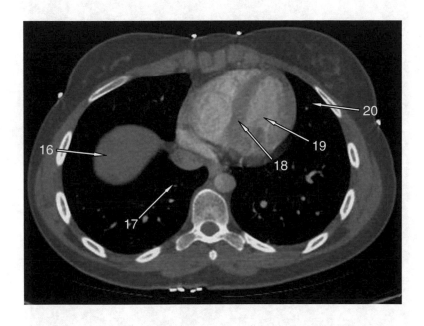

Questions	
16.	Name the structure labelled 16.
17.	Which segment and lobe is 17?
18.	Name the structure labelled 18.
19.	Name the structure labelled 19.
20.	Which segment and lobe is 20?

CT Head (3D Reconstruction)

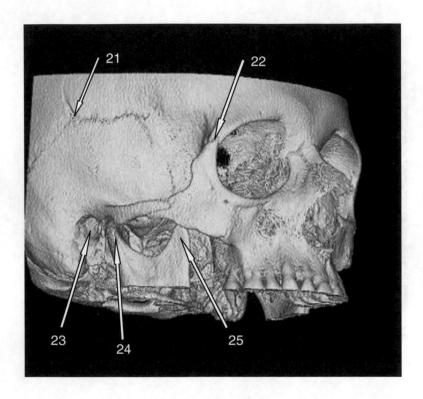

Questions	
21.	Name the structure labelled 21.
22.	Name the structure labelled 22.
23.	Name the structure labelled 23.
24.	Name the structure labelled 24.
25.	Name the structure labelled 25.

Hand Radiograph

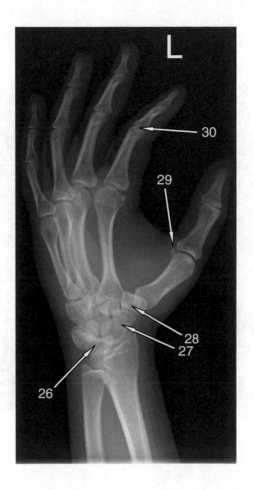

Questions	
26.	Name the structure labelled 26.
27.	Name the structure labelled 27.
28.	Name the structure labelled 28.
29.	Name the structure labelled 29.
30.	Name the structure labelled 30.

Ankle Radiograph

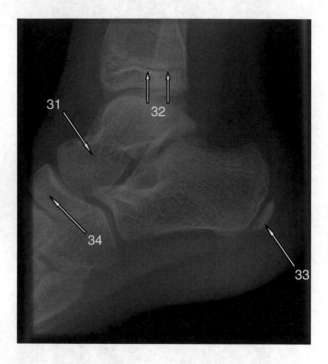

Questions	
31.	Name the structure labelled 31.
32.	Name the structure labelled 32.
33.	Name the structure labelled 33.
34.	Name the structure labelled 34.
35.	How old is this patient?

MRI Abdomen

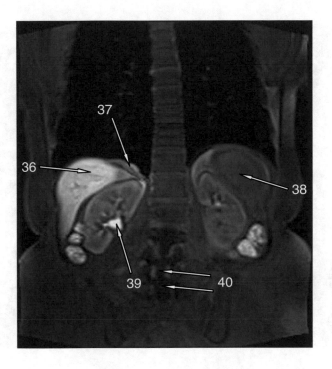

Questions	
36.	Name the structure labelled 36.
37.	Name the structure labelled 37.
38.	Name the structure labelled 38.
39.	Name the structure labelled 39.
40.	Name the structure labelled 40.

CT Abdomen

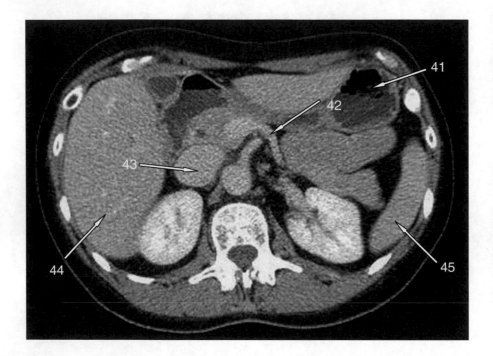

Questions	
41.	Name the structure labelled 41.
42.	Name the structure labelled 42.
43.	Name the structure labelled 43.
44.	Name the structure labelled 44.
45.	Name the structure labelled 45.

MRI Pelvis

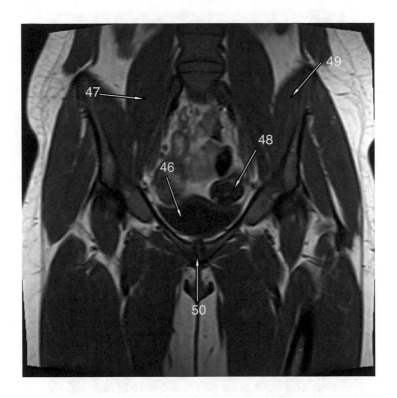

Questions	
46.	Name the structure labelled 46.
47.	Name the structure labelled 47.
48.	Name the structure labelled 48.
49.	Name the structure labelled 49.
50.	Name the structure labelled 50.

C-Spine Radiograph

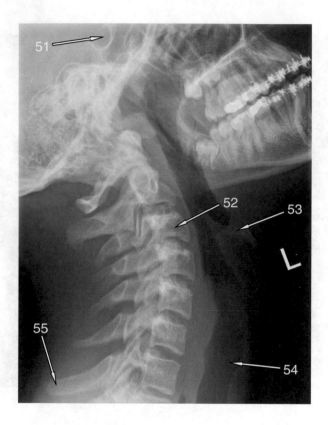

Questions	
51.	Name the structure labelled 51.
52.	What nerve root exits below 52?
53.	Name the structure labelled 53.
54.	Name the structure labelled 54.
55.	Name the structure labelled 55.

MR Angiogram

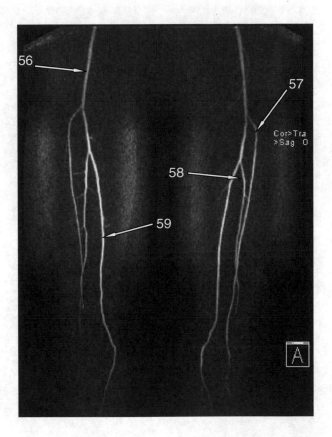

Questions	
56.	Name the structure labelled 56.
57.	Name the structure labelled 57.
58.	Name the structure labelled 58.
59.	Name the structure labelled 59.
60.	What vessel does vessel 57 become more distally?

IVU

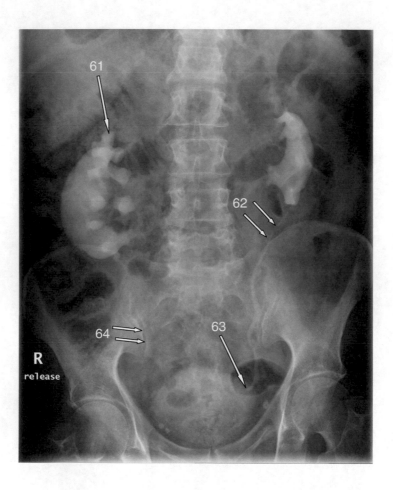

Questions	
61.	Name the structure labelled 61.
62.	Name the structure labelled 62.
63.	Name the structure labelled 63.
64.	Name the structure labelled 64.
65.	What anatomical variant is present?

MRI Brain

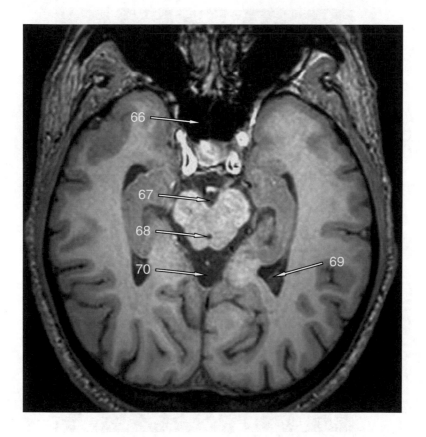

Questions	
66.	Name the structure labelled 66.
67.	Name the structure labelled 67.
68.	Name the structure labelled 68.
69.	Name the structure labelled 69.
70.	Name the structure labelled 70.

Ultrasound Abdomen

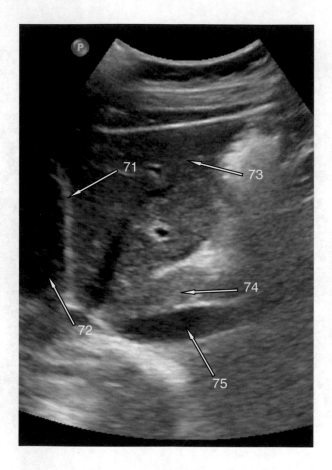

Questions	
71.	Name the structure labelled 71.
72.	Name the structure labelled 72.
73.	Name the structure labelled 73.
74.	Name the structure labelled 74.
75.	Name the structure labelled 75.

Urethrogram

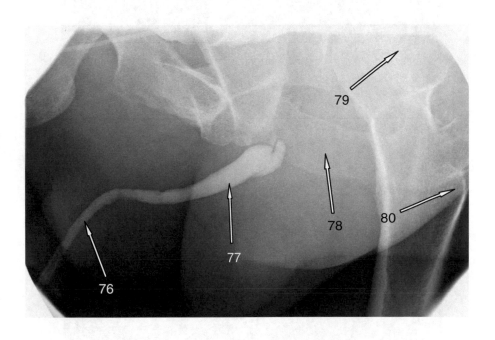

Questions	
76.	Name the structure labelled 76.
77.	Name the structure labelled 77.
78.	Name the structure labelled 78.
79.	Name the structure labelled 79.
80.	Name the structure labelled 80.

Shoulder Radiograph

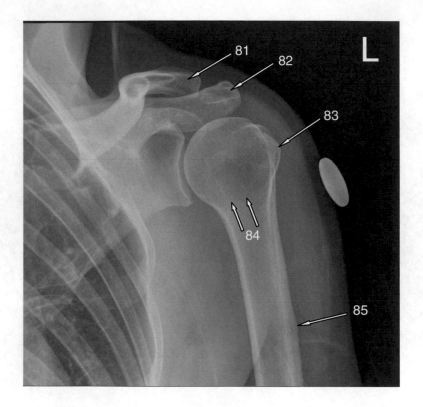

Questions	
81.	Name the structure labelled 81.
82.	Name the structure labelled 82.
83.	Name the structure labelled 83.
84.	Name the structure labelled 84.
85.	Name the structure labelled 85.

Foot Radiograph

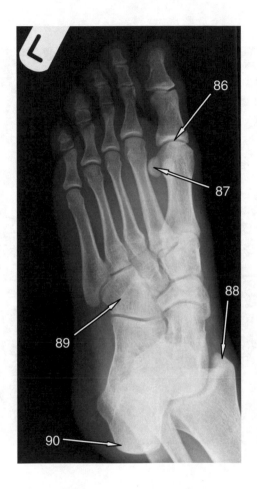

Questions	
86.	Name the structure labelled 86.
87.	Name the structure labelled 87.
88.	Name the structure labelled 88.
89.	Name the structure labelled 89.
90.	Name the structure labelled 90.

Chest Radiograph

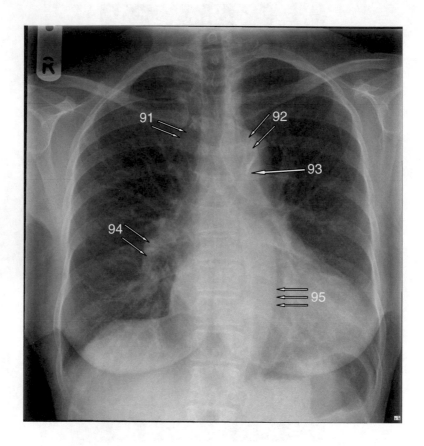

Questions	
91.	Name the structure labelled 91.
92.	Name the structure labelled 92.
93.	Name the structure labelled 93.
94.	Name the structure labelled 94.
95.	Name the structure labelled 95.

MRI Brain

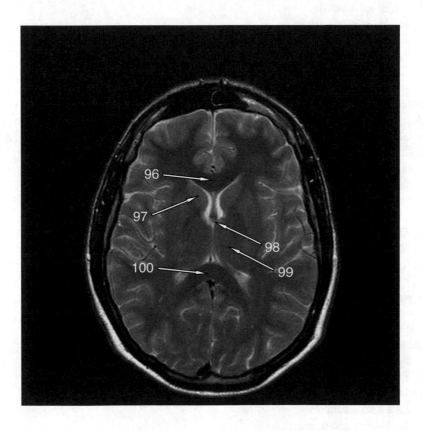

Questions	
96.	Name the structure labelled 96.
97.	Name the structure labelled 97.
98.	Name the structure labelled 98.
99.	Name the structure labelled 99.
100.	Name the structure labelled 100.

Test 3 Answers

MRI Head

1. Right optic nerve
2. Right abducens nerve
3. Right inferior concha/turbinate
4. Left inferior rectus muscle
5. Left temporalis muscle

Innervation of the muscles of the eye: *Lr6SO4*, *L*ateral *r*ectus cranial nerve VI (abducens nerve), *S*uperior *O*blique cranial nerve IV (trochlear nerve). The other muscles (superior, medial and inferior recti and inferior obliques) are supplied by cranial nerve III (oculomotor nerve).

Barium Enema

6. Caecum/caecal pole
7. Right iliac crest
8. Transverse colon
9. Descending colon
10. Left anterior superior iliac spine

Elbow Radiograph

11. Left shaft of ulna
12. Left tuberosity of radius
13. Left neck of radius
14. Left olecranon of ulna
15. Left triceps brachii muscle

Another possible question is what muscle inserts into 12? (Biceps brachii muscle)

CT Chest

16. Right hemidiaphragm (right lobe of liver)
17. Medial segment of right lower lobe
18. Interventricular septum
19. Left ventricular cavity
20. Lingula segment of left upper lobe

CT Head (3D Reconstruction)

21. Right pterion
22. Right fronto-zygomatic suture
23. Right external acoustic meatus of temporal bone
24. Right condyle of mandible
25. Right coronoid process mandible

3D reconstruction software is an easily available and useful tool; expect some similar cases in the exam.

Hand Radiograph

26. Left lunate bone
27. Left scaphoid bone
28. Left trapezium
29. Sesamoid bone at left thumb metacarpophalangeal joint
30. Proximal interphalangeal joint (PIPJ) of left index finger

Ankle Radiograph

31. Talus (neck of talus)
32. Distal tibial physeal line
33. Unfused calcaneus secondary ossification centre
34. Navicular bone
35. Between 5 years old and puberty

The calcaneus has two ossification centres. The posterior centre ossifies at age 5 and fuses at puberty.

MRI Abdomen

36. Right lobe of liver
37. Right hemidiaphragm
38. Spleen
39. Right renal pelvis
40. Thecal sac

The plane of this MRI section is such that the thecal sac is exposed in the lower lumbar segments.

CT Abdomen

41. Stomach
42. Splenic vein
43. Inferior vena cava
44. Right lobe of the liver (segment VI)
45. Spleen

Look for the tadpole sign of the splenic vein (tail) going to join the inferior mesenteric vein to form the portal vein (head).

MRI Pelvis

46. Urinary bladder
47. Right psoas major muscle
48. Sigmoid colon
49. Left iliacus muscle
50. Symphysis pubis

C-Spine Radiograph

51. Pituitary fossa or sella turcica
52. C4 nerve root
53. Hyoid bone (body of)
54. Trachea
55. C7 spinous process

Remember that there are eight cervical nerves and seven cervical vertebrae. The first seven cervical nerves emerge above the named vertebrae (above C3=C3 nerve root). The C8 nerve root exits below the C7 vertebra.

MR Angiogram

56. Right superficial femoral artery
57. Left anterior tibial artery
58. Left peroneal artery
59. Right posterior tibial artery
60. Left dorsalis pedis artery

The anterior tibial artery is the first lateral branch from the popliteal artery.

IVU

61. Right major calyx (upper pole)
62. Left ureter
63. Left vesicoureteric junction
64. Right sacroiliac joint
65. Horseshoe kidney

Horseshoe kidney is the most common renal fusion anomaly. In 90 % of cases fusion occurs at the lower pole (as in this example). Note the malrotated collecting systems (renal pelvis laterally, calyces medially).

MRI Brain

66. Sphenoidal sinus
67. Interpeduncular cistern
68. Aqueduct of Sylvius
69. Choroid plexus in trigone of left lateral ventricle
70. Quadrigeminal cistern

The corpora quadrigemina is made up of the superior and inferior colliculi. The quadrigeminal cistern is the subarachnoid space posterior to it. It contains the confluence of veins which form the great cerebral vein of Galen.

Ultrasound Abdomen

71. Diaphragm
72. Right lung
73. Left lobe of liver
74. Caudate lobe of liver
75. Inferior Vena Cava

This is a standard longitudinal (sagittal) view through the upper abdomen showing the caudate lobe between the left lobe of liver and the IVC. The IVC traverses the central tendon of the diaphragm to the right of midline. The diaphragm is echo bright.

Urethrogram

76. Penile urethra
77. Bulbous urethra
78. Inferior pubic ramus
79. Head of femur
80. Greater trochanter of femur

Shoulder Radiograph

81. Left clavicle
82. Acromion process (of left scapula)
83. Left greater tuberosity of humerus
84. Left surgical neck of humerus
85. Left deltoid tuberosity of humerus

Foot Radiograph

86. Left 1st metatarsophalangeal joint
87. Left sesamoid bone in flexor hallucis brevis tendon
88. Medial malleolus of left tibia
89. Left cuboid
90. Left calcaneus

Chest Radiograph

91. Manubrium
92. Aortic knuckle
93. Aortopulmonary window
94. Interlobar artery
95. Descending thoracic aorta

MRI Brain

96. Genu of corpus callosum
97. Head of right caudate nucleus
98. Left interventricular foramen of Monro
99. Left thalamus
100. Splenium of corpus callosum

Test 4

4

(You have 90 minutes to complete 100 questions)

CT Abdomen

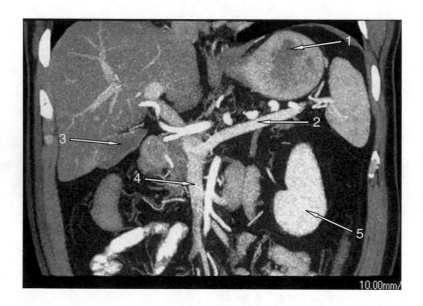

Questions	
1.	Name the structure labelled 1.
2.	Name the structure labelled 2.
3.	Name the structure labelled 3.
4.	Name the structure labelled 4.
5.	Name the structure labelled 5.

CT Head (3D Reconstruction)

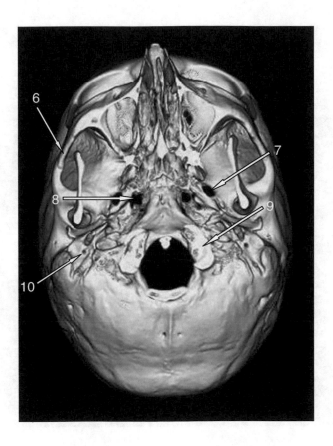

Questions	
6.	Name the structure labelled 6.
7.	Name the structure labelled 7.
8.	What structure passes through 8?
9.	Name the structure labelled 9.
10.	Name the structure labelled 10.

MRI Ankle

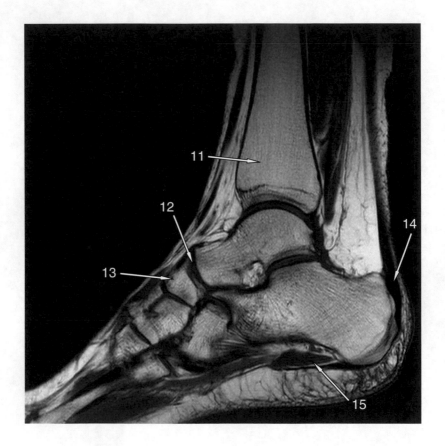

Questions	
11.	Name the structure labelled 11.
12.	Name the structure labelled 12.
13.	Name the structure labelled 13.
14.	Name the structure labelled 14.
15.	Name the structure labelled 15.

Ultrasound Abdomen

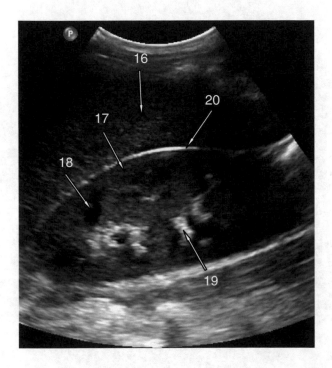

Questions	
16.	Name the structure labelled 16.
17.	Name the structure labelled 17.
18.	Name the structure labelled 18.
19.	Name the structure labelled 19.
20.	Name the potential space labelled 20.

Barium Meal

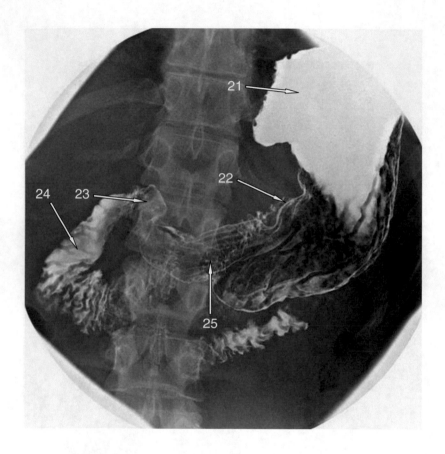

Questions	
21.	Name the structure labelled 21.
22.	Name the structure labelled 22.
23.	Name the structure labelled 23.
24.	Name the structure labelled 24.
25.	Name the structure labelled 25.

IVU

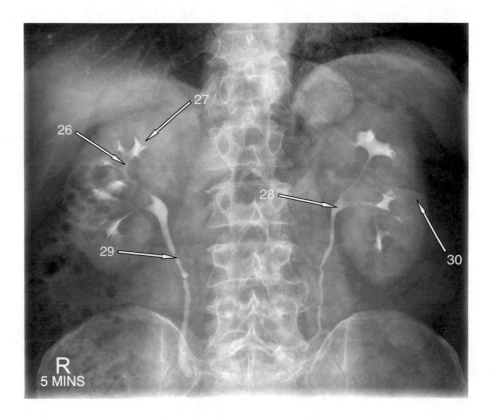

Questions	
26.	Name the structure labelled 26.
27.	Name the structure labelled 27.
28.	Name the structure labelled 28.
29.	Name the structure labelled 29.
30.	Name the structure labelled 30.

Skull Radiograph

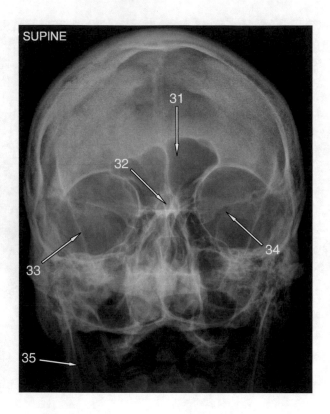

Questions	
31.	Name the structure labelled 31.
32.	Name the structure labelled 32.
33.	Name the structure labelled 33.
34.	Name the structure labelled 34.
35.	Name the structure labelled 35.

CT Lumbar Spine (3D Reconstruction)

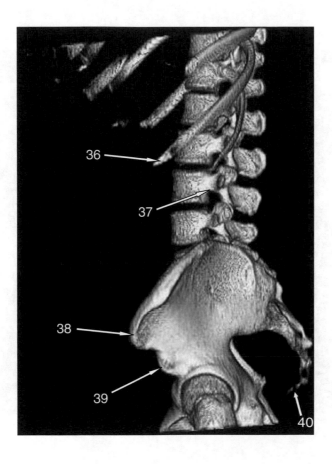

Questions	
36.	Name the structure labelled 36.
37.	Name the structure labelled 37.
38.	Name the structure labelled 38.
39.	Name the structure labelled 39.
40.	Name the structure labelled 40.

CT Abdomen

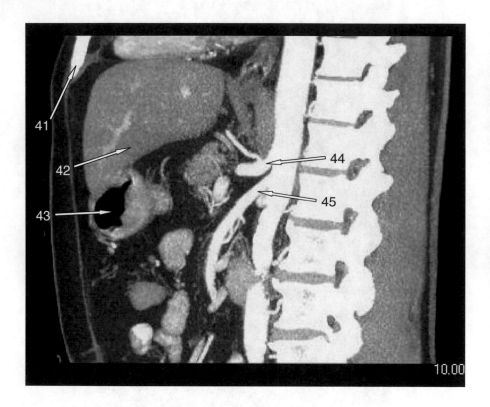

Questions	
41.	Name the structure labelled 41.
42.	Name the structure labelled 42.
43.	Name the structure labelled 43.
44.	Name the structure labelled 44.
45.	Name the structure labelled 45.

MRI Brain

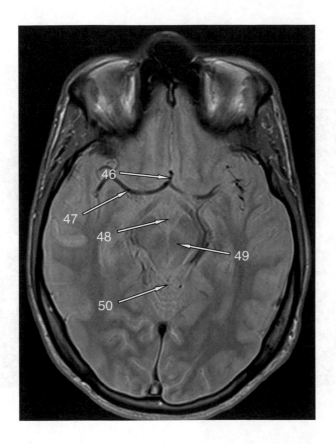

Questions	
46.	Name the structure labelled 46.
47.	Name the structure labelled 47.
48.	Name the structure labelled 48.
49.	Name the structure labelled 49.
50.	Name the structure labelled 50.

CT Abdomen

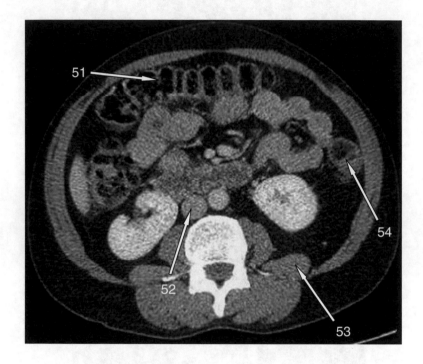

Questions	
51.	Name the structure labelled 51.
52.	Name the structure labelled 52.
53.	Name the structure labelled 53.
54.	Name the structure labelled 54.
55.	What normal variant is present?

MRI Ankle

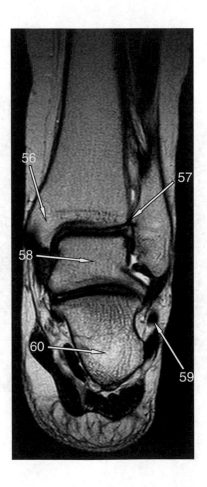

Questions	
56.	Name the structure labelled 56.
57.	Name the structure labelled 57.
58.	Name the structure labelled 58.
59.	Name the structure labelled 59.
60.	Name the structure labelled 60.

CT Chest

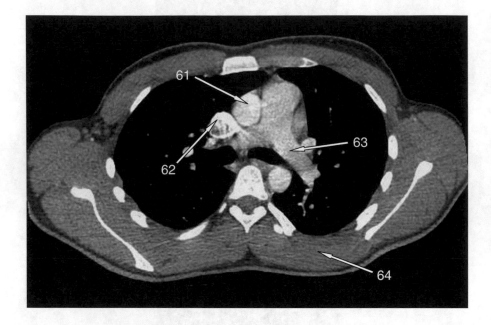

Questions	
61.	Name the structure labelled 61.
62.	Name the structure labelled 62.
63.	Name the structure labelled 63.
64.	Name the structure labelled 64.
65.	What vertebral level is this axial slice?

CT Sinuses

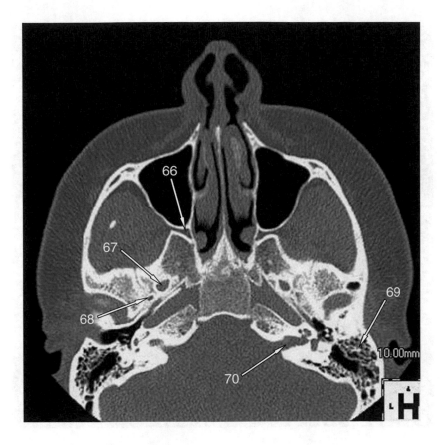

Questions	
66.	Name the structure labelled 66.
67.	Name the structure labelled 67.
68.	Name the structure labelled 68.
69.	Name the structure labelled 69.
70.	Name the structure labelled 70.

CT Abdomen

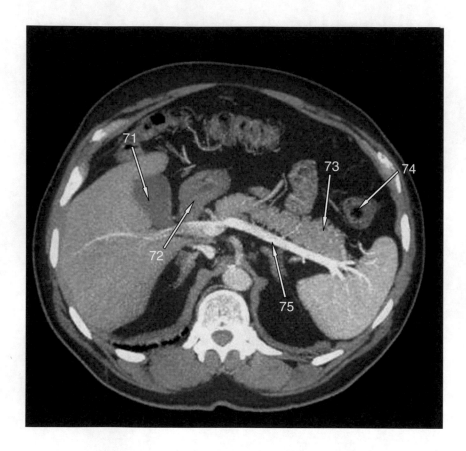

Questions	
71.	Name the structure labelled 71.
72.	Name the structure labelled 72.
73.	Name the structure labelled 73.
74.	Name the structure labelled 74.
75.	Name the structure labelled 75.

CT Abdomen

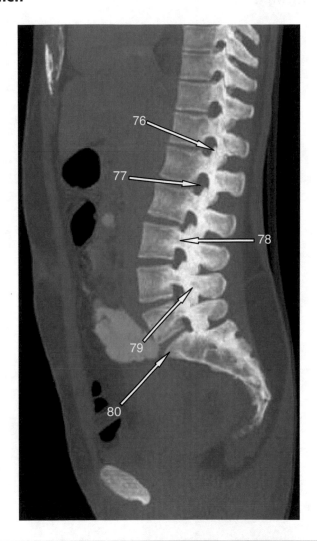

Questions	
76.	Name the structure labelled 76.
77.	Name the structure labelled 77.
78.	Name the structure labelled 78.
79.	Name the structure labelled 79.
80.	Name the structure labelled 80.

Ankle Radiograph

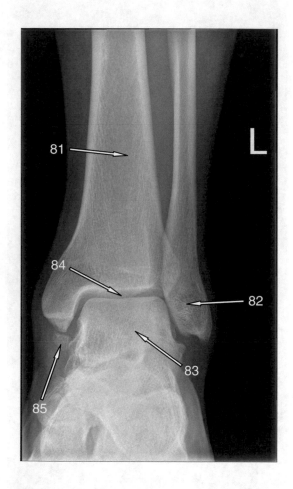

Questions	
81.	Name the structure labelled 81.
82.	Name the structure labelled 82.
83.	Name the structure labelled 83.
84.	Name the structure labelled 84.
85.	Name the structure labelled 85.

Hysterosalpingogram

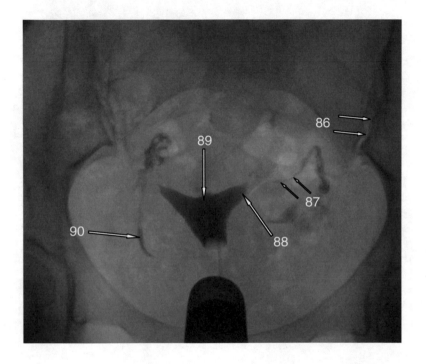

Questions	
86.	Name the structure labelled 86.
87.	Name the structure labelled 87.
88.	Name the structure labelled 88.
89.	Name the structure labelled 89.
90.	Name the structure labelled 90.

Ultrasound Testes

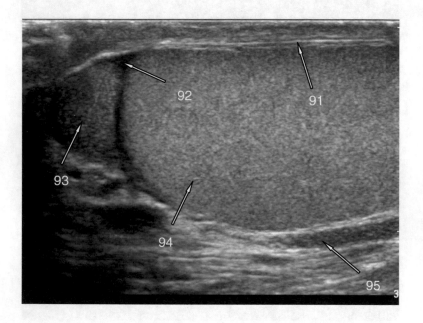

Questions	
91.	Name the structure labelled 91.
92.	Name the structure labelled 92.
93.	Name the structure labelled 93.
94.	Name the structure labelled 94.
95.	Name the structure labelled 95.

CT Sinuses

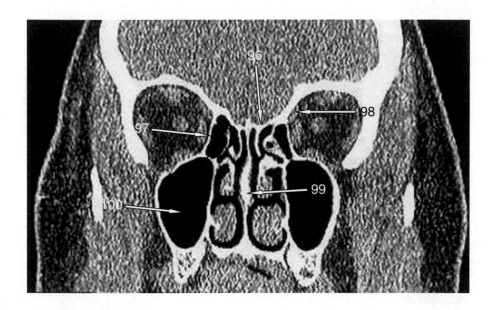

Questions	
96.	Name the structure labelled 96.
97.	Name the structure labelled 97.
98.	Name the structure labelled 98.
99.	Name the structure labelled 99.
100.	Name the structure labelled 100.

Test 4 Answers

CT Abdomen

1. Stomach
2. Splenic vein
3. Gall bladder
4. Superior mesenteric vein
5. Left kidney

The portal vein is formed by the union of the splenic vein and the superior mesenteric vein behind the neck of the pancreas. It drains blood from the lower 1st/3rd of the oesophagus to halfway down the anal canal.

CT Head (3D Reconstruction)

6. Right zygomatic arch
7. Left foramen ovale
8. Right internal carotid artery
9. Left occipital condyle
10. Right stylomastoid foramen

The foramen lacerum transmits the internal carotid artery (as well as the vessels and nerve of the pterygoid canal).

MRI Ankle

11. Tibia (distal metaphysis of)
12. Talonavicular joint
13. Navicular bone
14. Achilles' tendon
15. Abductor digiti minimi muscle

Ultrasound Abdomen

16. Right lobe of liver
17. Renal cortex of right kidney
18. Medullary pyramid of right kidney
19. Renal sinus fat of right kidney
20. Morrison's pouch

Morrison's pouch lies between the posterior surface of the liver and the right kidney. In the supine position it is the most dependent of the peritoneal spaces, and free fluid will therefore often pool here.

Barium Meal

21. Gastric Fundus (barium within)
22. Lesser curvature of stomach
23. Duodenal cap (D1 segment)
24. 2nd part of duodenum (D2 segment)
25. Antrum of stomach

IVU

26. Right minor calyx (upper pole)
27. Right renal papilla
28. Left renal pelvis
29. Right ureter
30. Left renal cortex

The renal papilla drains into a minor calyx which then drains into a major calyx, which in turn drains into the renal pelvis.

Skull Radiograph

31. Left frontal sinus
32. Crista galli
33. Right innominate line
34. Left superior orbital fissure
35. Right ramus of mandible

The innominate line is formed by the lateral greater wing of sphenoid.
    The superior orbital fissure transmits cranial nerves III, IV, V (ophthalmic division), VI and sympathetic nerves.

CT Lumbar Spine (3D Reconstruction)

36. Left 11th rib (tip of)
37. Left pedicle of L3 vertebra
38. Left anterior superior iliac spine
39. Left anterior inferior iliac spine
40. Coccyx

To identify the level of a vertebra, count down from T12 (origin of 12th rib).
    The coccyx is formed from four fused vertebrae.

CT Abdomen

41. Xiphisternum
42. Liver
43. Stomach
44. Coeliac axis
45. Superior mesenteric artery

Aortic branches in the abdomen:

T12 – Coeliac trunk arises.
L1 – Superior mesenteric.
L2 – Renal arteries.
L3 – Inferior mesenteric artery.
L4 – Aorta divides into right and left common iliac arteries.
L5/S1 – Common iliac arteries divide into internal and external iliac arteries.

MRI Brain

46. Left anterior cerebral artery
47. Right middle cerebral artery
48. Interpeduncular cistern
49. Left red nucleus
50. Quadrigeminal cistern

CT Abdomen

51. Transverse colon
52. Inferior vena cava
53. Left quadratus lumborum muscle
54. Descending colon
55. Malrotated right kidney

Note how the right renal pelvis faces laterally.

MRI Ankle

56. Medial malleolus of tibia
57. Inferior tibiofibular ligament
58. Talus
59. Tendon of peroneus brevis muscle
60. Calcaneum

CT Chest

61. Ascending thoracic aorta
62. Superior vena cava
63. Left main pulmonary artery
64. Left trapezius
65. T5–T7

Bifurcation of carina occurs at T5–T7 level.

CT Sinuses

66. Right pterygopalatine fossa
67. Right foramen ovale
68. Right foramen spinosum
69. Left mastoid air cells
70. Left internal auditory meatus

The internal auditory meatus/internal acoustic meatus is a canal in the petrous part of the *temporal bone*. The VII and VIII cranial nerves enter here.

CT Abdomen

71. Gall bladder
72. 2nd part duodenum (D2 segment)
73. Tail of pancreas
74. Splenic flexure of large intestine (descending colon)
75. Splenic vein

CT Abdomen

76. Superior articular process of L1 vertebra
77. L1/L2 intervertebral foramen
78. Pedicle L3 vertebra
79. Pars interarticularis of L4 vertebra
80. Sacral promontory

The pars interarticularis is the part of the lamina between the superior and inferior articular facets. The transverse processes are formed at the junction of the pedicle and lamina. The laminae fuse to form the spinous process posteriorly.

Ankle Radiograph

81. Left diaphysis tibia
82. Left lateral malleolus (of fibula)
83. Left talus
84. Left tibio-talar joint
85. Unfused epiphysis left medial malleolus (of tibia)

Hysterosalpingogram

86. Left sacroiliac joint
87. Left Isthmus of uterine tube
88. Left cornu of uterus
89. Fundus of uterus
90. Free peritoneal spillage

This is a hysterosalpingogram (HSG). The metal density object at the bottom of the image is a vaginal speculum. One can also see an inflated balloon just above the cervix.

Ultrasound Testes

91. Tunica albuginea
92. Fluid within scrotal sac
93. Epididymal head
94. Testis
95. Body of epididymis

CT Sinuses

96. Left cribriform plate
97. Right lamina papyracea
98. Left superior oblique muscle
99. Nasal septum
100. Right maxillary sinus

The lamina papyracea/orbital lamina forms a large part of the medial wall of the orbit and is part of the ethmoid bone. Its name refers to the fact that it is paper thin and fractures easily.

Test 5

(You have 90 minutes to complete 100 questions)

P. Borg et al., *Radiological Anatomy for FRCR Part 1*,
DOI 10.1007/978-3-642-41166-3_5, © Springer-Verlag Berlin Heidelberg 2014

ERCP

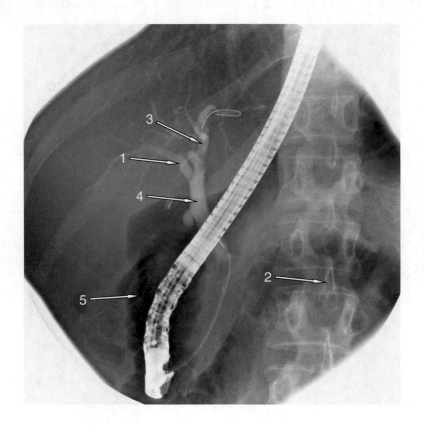

Questions	
1.	Name the structure labelled 1.
2.	Name the structure labelled 2.
3.	Name the structure labelled 3.
4.	Name the structure labelled 4.
5.	Name the structure labelled 5.

MRA

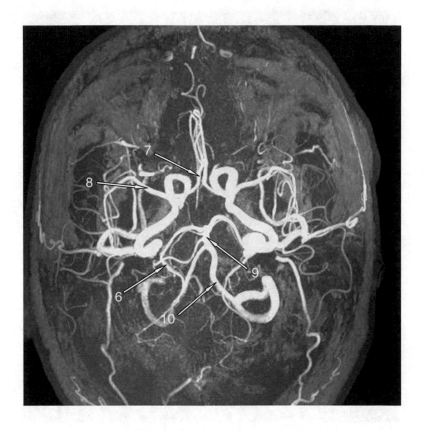

Questions	
6.	Name the structure labelled 6.
7.	Name the structure labelled 7.
8.	Name the structure labelled 8.
9.	Name the structure labelled 9.
10.	Name the structure labelled 10.

CT Head

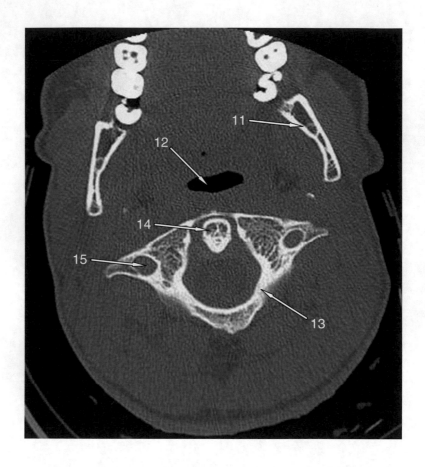

Questions	
11.	Name the structure labelled 11.
12.	Name the structure labelled 12.
13.	Name the structure that runs in the groove labelled 13.
14.	Name the structure labelled 14.
15.	Name the structure labelled 15.

MRCP

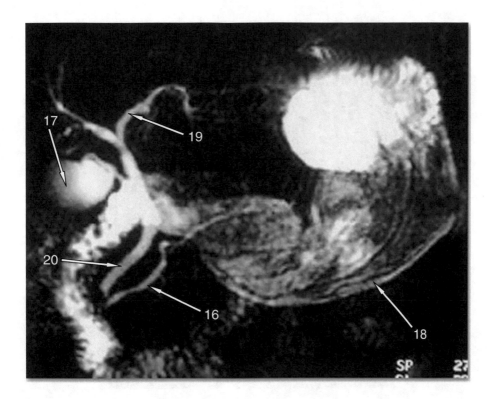

Questions	
16.	Name the structure labelled 16.
17.	Name the structure labelled 17.
18.	Name the structure labelled 18.
19.	Name the structure labelled 19.
20.	Name the structure labelled 20.

MRA

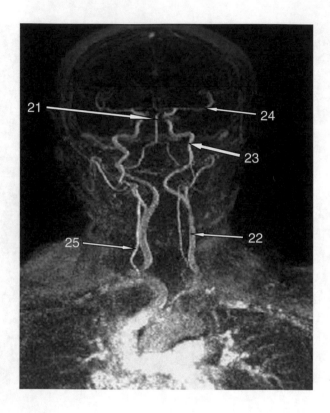

Questions	
21.	Name the structure labelled 21.
22.	Name the structure labelled 22.
23.	Name the structure labelled 23.
24.	Name the structure labelled 24.
25.	Name the structure labelled 25.

Ultrasound Pelvis

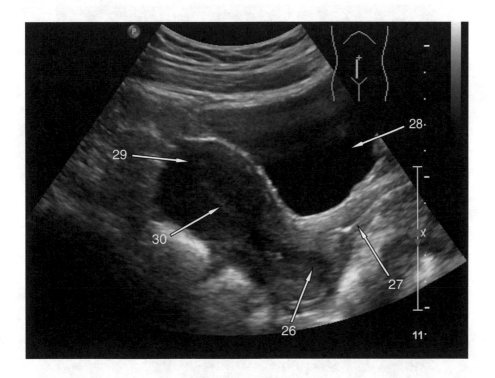

Questions	
26.	Name the structure labelled 26.
27.	Name the structure labelled 27.
28.	Name the structure labelled 28.
29.	Name the structure labelled 29.
30.	Name the structure labelled 30.

MRI Head

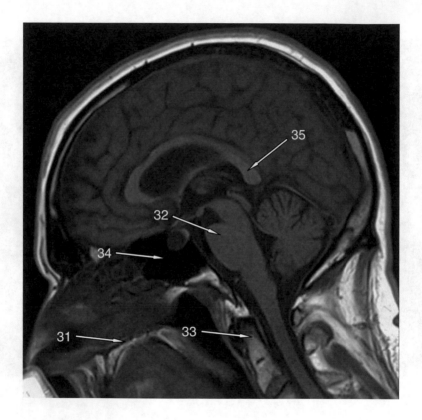

Questions	
31.	Name the structure labelled 31.
32.	Name the structure labelled 32.
33.	Name the structure labelled 33.
34.	Name the structure labelled 34.
35.	Name the structure labelled 35.

Orthopantomogram

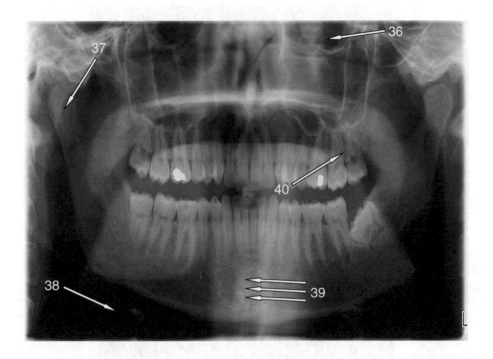

Questions	
36.	Name the structure labelled 36.
37.	Name the structure labelled 37.
38.	Name the structure labelled 38.
39.	Name the structure labelled 39.
40.	Name the structure that opens into the buccal cavity at 40.

MRI Knee

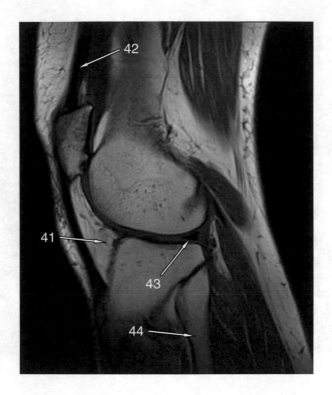

Questions	
41.	Name the structure labelled 41.
42.	Name the structure labelled 42.
43.	Name the structure labelled 43.
44.	Name the structure labelled 44.
45.	Name the structure that can be damaged if a fracture occurs at 44.

Ultrasound Abdomen

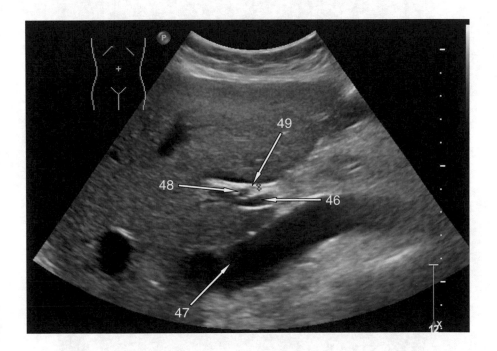

Questions	
46.	Name the structure labelled 46.
47.	Name the structure labelled 47.
48.	Name the structure labelled 48.
49.	Name the structure labelled 49.
50.	Name the opening into the lesser sac whose anterior margin is formed by structures 46, 48 and 49.

CT Pelvis

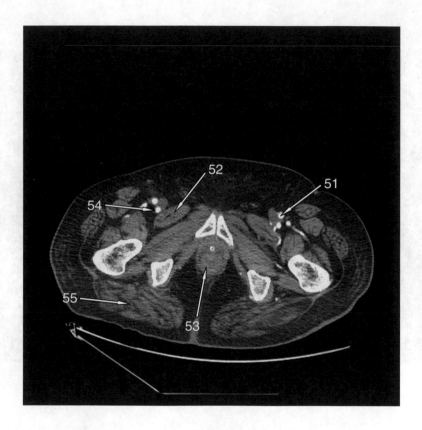

Questions	
51.	Name the structure labelled 51.
52.	Name the structure labelled 52.
53.	Name the structure labelled 53.
54.	Name the structure labelled 54.
55.	Name the structure labelled 55.

Ultrasound Neck

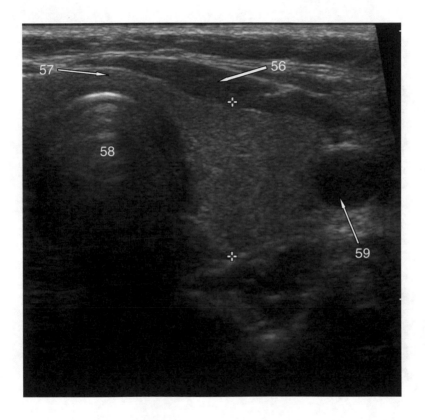

Questions	
56.	Name the structure labelled 56.
57.	Name the structure labelled 57.
58.	Name the structure labelled 58.
59.	Name the structure labelled 59.
60.	Name the structure into which 59 drains into?

CT Abdomen

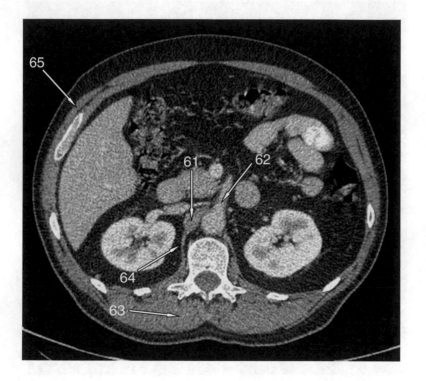

Questions	
61.	Name the structure labelled 61.
62.	Name the structure labelled 62.
63.	Name the structure labelled 63.
64.	Name the structure labelled 64.
65.	Name the structure labelled 65.

CT Chest

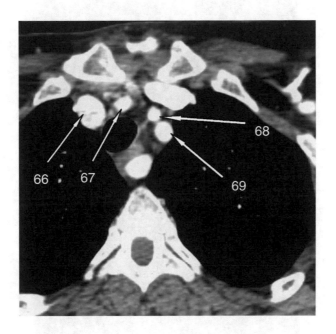

Questions	
66.	Name the structure labelled 66.
67.	Name the structure labelled 67.
68.	Name the structure labelled 68.
69.	Name the structure labelled 69.
70.	Name the anatomical variant.

Elbow Radiograph

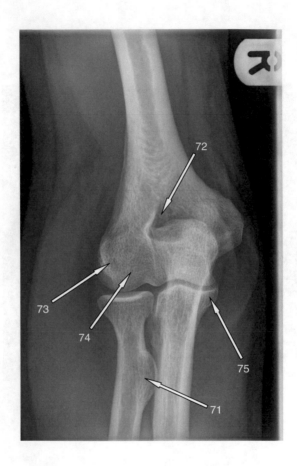

Questions	
71.	Name the structure labelled 71.
72.	Name the structure labelled 72.
73.	Name the structure labelled 73.
74.	Name the structure labelled 74.
75.	Name the structure labelled 75.

Shoulder Radiograph

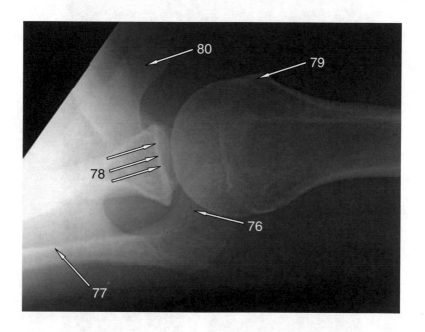

Questions	
76.	Name the structure labelled 76.
77.	Name the structure labelled 77.
78.	Name the structure labelled 78.
79.	Name the structure labelled 79.
80.	Name the structure labelled 80.

Abdominal Radiograph

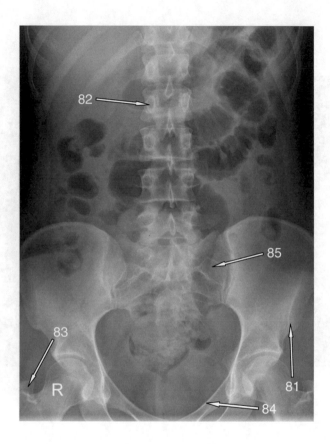

Questions	
81.	Name the structure labelled 81.
82.	Name the structure labelled 82.
83.	Name the structure labelled 83.
84.	Name the structure labelled 84.
85.	Name the structure labelled 85.

Cervical Spine Radiograph

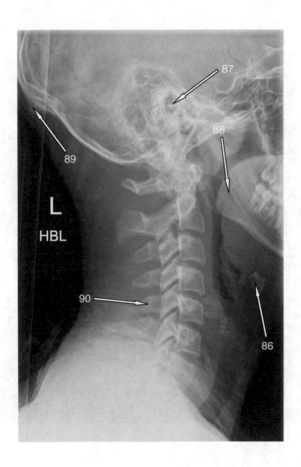

Questions	
86.	Name the structure labelled 86.
87.	Name the structure labelled 87.
88.	Name the structure labelled 88.
89.	Name the structure labelled 89.
90.	Name the structure labelled 90.

DSA

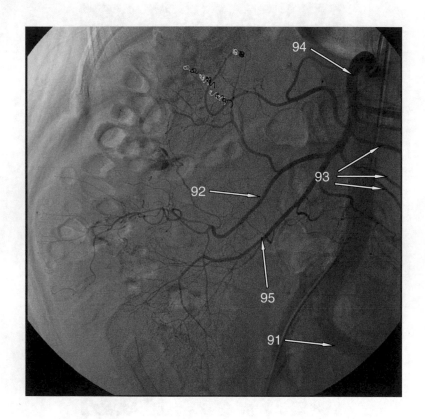

Questions	
91.	Name the structure labelled 91.
92.	Name the structure labelled 92.
93.	Name the structure labelled 93.
94.	Name the structure labelled 94.
95.	Name the structure labelled 95.

Barium Meal

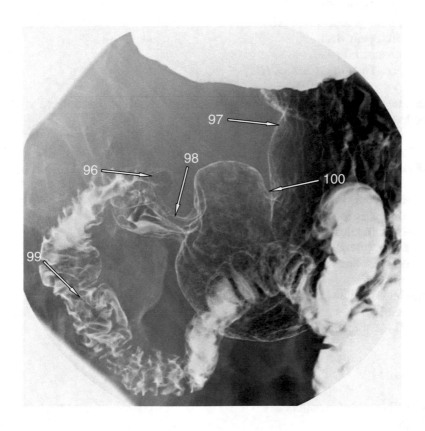

Questions	
96.	Name the structure labelled 96.
97.	Name the structure labelled 97.
98.	Name the structure labelled 98.
99.	Name the structure labelled 99.
100.	Name the structure labelled 100.

Test 5 Answers

ERCP

1. Right hepatic duct
2. Spinous process L2 vertebra
3. Left hepatic duct
4. Common bile duct
5. Second part of duodenum (D2)

The ampulla of Vater is located in the posteromedial wall of the second part of the duodenum, which is selectively cannulated during ERCP.

MRA

6. Right posterior cerebral artery
7. Right anterior cerebral artery
8. Right middle cerebral artery
9. Basilar artery
10. Left vertebral artery

The Circle of Willis is an anastomosis between right and left internal carotid arteries, their branches and the posterior cerebral arteries. It is complete in 90 %, and there is variation of at least one vessel in around 60 %.

CT Head

11. Left ramus of mandible
12. Oropharynx
13. Left vertebral artery
14. Odontoid process (dens) of C2 (axis) vertebra
15. Right transverse foramen (foramen transversarium) of C1 (atlas) vertebra

At C1, the vertebral artery lies in the groove on the upper surface of the posterior arch of the atlas before entering the foramen magnum.

MRCP

16. Main pancreatic duct (of Wirsung)
17. Gallbladder
18. Greater curvature of stomach
19. Left hepatic duct
20. Common bile duct

MRA

21. Basilar artery
22. Left common carotid artery
23. Left internal carotid artery
24. Left middle cerebral artery
25. Left vertebral artery

Ultrasound Pelvis

26. Cervix
27. Vagina
28. Bladder
29. Uterine fundus
30. Endometrium

This is a longitudinal scan of the female pelvis. The cervix usually lies in the mid-line and the uterus may lie obliquely to either side. The endometrium is seen as a thin high-level echo on this image as a long white stripe. The normal endometrial thickness in the postmenopausal woman should be less than 3 mm.

MRI Head

31. Hard palate
32. Pons
33. Odontoid process of C2 (axis) vertebrae
34. Sphenoid sinus
35. Splenium of corpus callosum

Orthopantomogram

36. Left maxillary sinus
37. Right condyle of mandible
38. Hyoid bone
39. Symphysis menti
40. Parotid duct

This is an orthopantomogram – a panoramic image of dental arches, mandible, temporomandibular joints and lower maxilla.

MRI Knee

41. Hoffa's fat pad
42. Quadriceps tendon
43. Lateral meniscus
44. Neck of fibula
45. Common peroneal nerve

As the fibula is visible in this image, one can deduce that the meniscus demonstrated is the lateral meniscus. The common peroneal nerve winds around the head of the fibula and is prone to damage resulting in loss of dorsiflexion (foot drop).

Abdominal Ultrasound

46. Portal vein
47. Inferior vena cava
48. Hepatic artery
49. Common bile duct
50. Epiploic foramen

CT Pelvis

51. Left superficial femoral artery
52. Right pectineus muscle
53. Rectum
54. Right profunda femoris artery
55. Right gluteus maximus

This axial CT is at the level of the bifurcation of the CFA. Profunda (deep) femoral artery gives off the medial and lateral circumflex arteries and perforating branches to the deep muscles of the thigh.

Ultrasound Neck

56. Left sternomastoid muscle
57. Thyroid isthmus
58. Trachea
59. Left Internal jugular vein
60. Left brachiocephalic vein

CT Abdomen

61. Inferior vena cava
62. Superior mesenteric artery
63. Right erector spinae muscle
64. Right crus of diaphragm
65. Right external oblique muscle

CT Chest

66. Right Brachiocephalic vein
67. Right common carotid artery
68. Left common carotid artery
69. Left subclavian artery
70. Aberrant origin of right subclavian artery

This anatomical variant is also known as arteria lusoria and is the most common intrathoracic abnormality of the aortic arch, with an incidence of 1–2 %.

Elbow Radiograph

71. Tuberosity of right radius
72. Olecranon fossa of right humerus
73. Lateral epicondyle of right humerus
74. Capitellum of right humerus
75. Coronoid process of right ulna

Shoulder Radiograph

76. Acromion process of scapula
77. Spine of scapula
78. Glenoid fossa
79. Greater tuberosity of humerus
80. Coracoid process of scapula

The coracoid process is the most anterior part of the scapula. This should help you identify the other features on this image.

Abdominal Radiograph

81. Left anterior inferior iliac spine
82. Right pedicle of L2 vertebra
83. Greater trochanter of right femur
84. Left superior pubic ramus
85. Left ala of sacrum

Cervical Spine Radiograph

86. Hyoid bone
87. External auditory meatus
88. Angle of mandible
89. External occipital protuberance
90. Spinous process of C5 vertebra

DSA

91. Left common iliac artery
92. Right colic artery
93. Jejunal branches of SMA
94. Superior mesenteric artery
95. Ileocolic artery

The superior mesenteric artery originates at the level of L1. (Coeliac artery = T12, IMA = L2)

Barium Meal

96. Duodenal cap (1st part of duodenum)
97. Lesser curve of stomach
98. Pylorus
99. Second part of duodenum
100. Incisura angularis of lesser curve of stomach

Test 6

(You have 90 minutes to complete 100 questions)

P. Borg et al., *Radiological Anatomy for FRCR Part 1*,
DOI 10.1007/978-3-642-41166-3_6, © Springer-Verlag Berlin Heidelberg 2014

Cervical Spine Radiograph

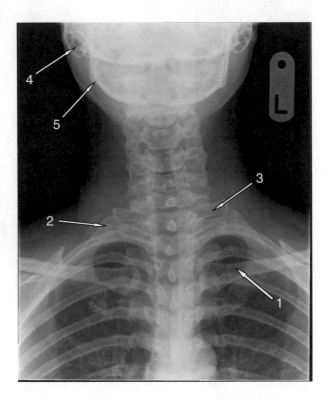

Questions	
1.	Name the structure labelled 1.
2.	Name the structure labelled 2.
3.	Name the structure labelled 3.
4.	Name the structure labelled 4.
5.	Name the structure labelled 5.

DSA

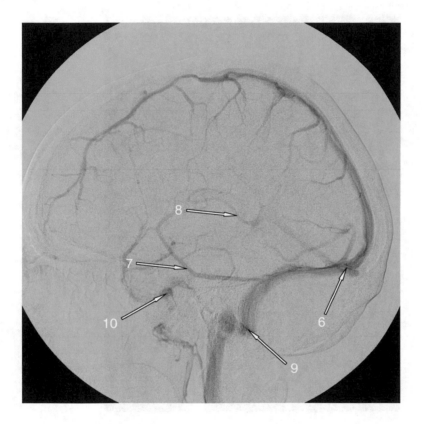

Questions	
6.	Name the structure labelled 6.
7.	Name the structure labelled 7.
8.	Name the structure labelled 8.
9.	Name the structure labelled 9.
10.	Name the structure labelled 10.

MRI Head

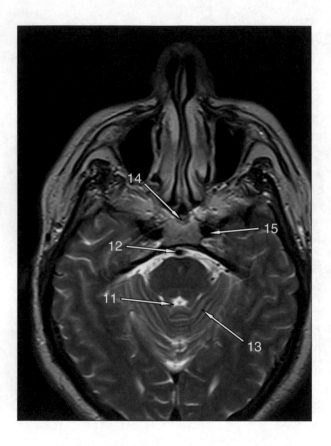

Questions	
11.	Name the structure labelled 11.
12.	Name the structure labelled 12.
13.	Name the structure labelled 13.
14.	Name the structure labelled 14.
15.	Name the structure labelled 15.

MRI Pelvis

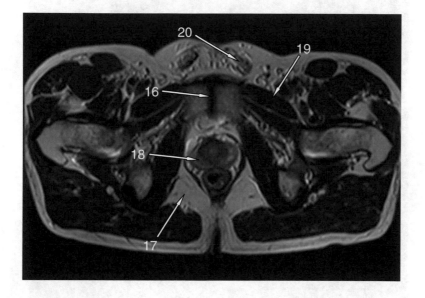

Questions	
16.	Name the structure labelled 16.
17.	Name the structure labelled 17.
18.	Name the structure labelled 18.
19.	Name the structure labelled 19.
20.	Name the structure labelled 20.

MRI Chest

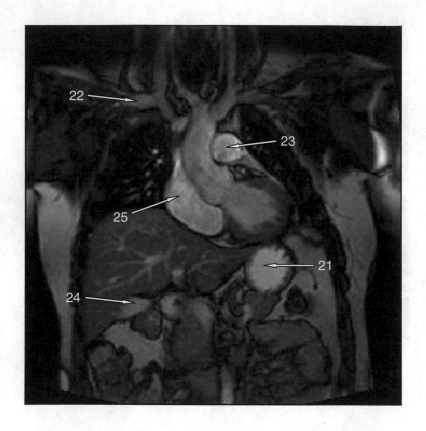

Questions	
21.	Name the structure labelled 21.
22.	Name the structure labelled 22.
23.	Name the structure labelled 23.
24.	Name the structure labelled 24.
25.	Name the structure labelled 25.

CT Heart

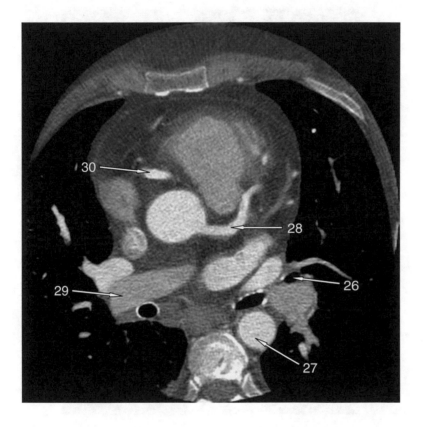

Questions	
26.	Name the structure labelled 26.
27.	Name the structure labelled 27.
28.	Name the structure labelled 28.
29.	Name the structure labelled 29.
30.	Name the structure labelled 30.

DSA

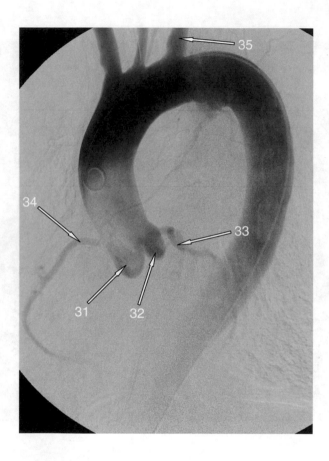

Questions	
31.	Name the structure labelled 31.
32.	Name the structure labelled 32.
33.	Name the structure labelled 33.
34.	Name the structure labelled 34.
35.	Name the structure labelled 35.

Ultrasound Abdomen

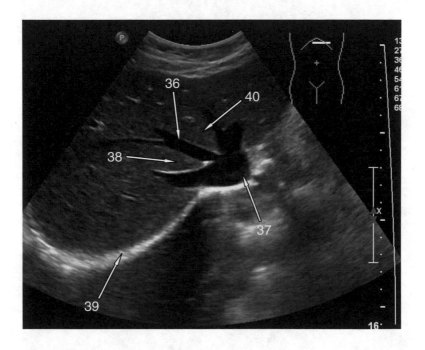

Questions	
36.	Name the structure labelled 36.
37.	Name the structure labelled 37.
38.	Name the structure labelled 38.
39.	Name the structure labelled 39.
40.	Name the structure labelled 40.

Barium Enema

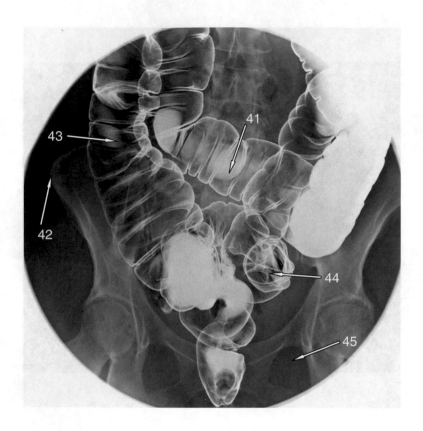

Questions	
41.	Name the structure labelled 41.
42.	Name the structure labelled 42.
43.	Name the structure labelled 43.
44.	Name the structure labelled 44.
45.	Name the structure labelled 45.

CT Head

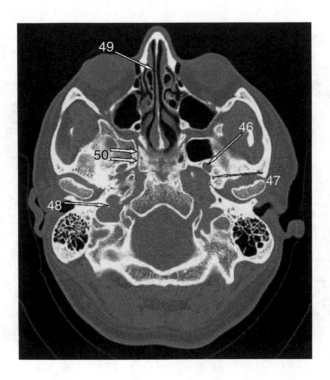

Questions	
46.	Name the structure labelled 46.
47.	Name the structure labelled 47.
48.	Name the structure labelled 48.
49.	Name the structure labelled 49.
50.	Name the structure labelled 50.

Ultrasound Abdomen

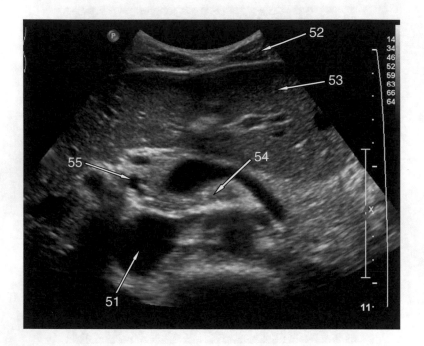

Questions	
51.	Name the structure labelled 51.
52.	Name the structure labelled 52.
53.	Name the structure labelled 53.
54.	Name the structure labelled 54.
55.	Name the structure labelled 55.

CT Chest

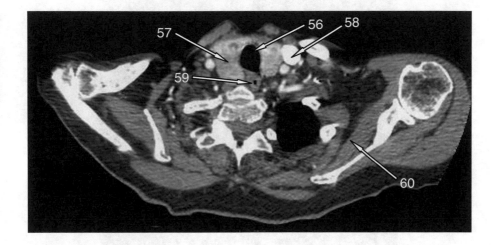

Questions	
56.	Name the structure labelled 56.
57.	Name the structure labelled 57.
58.	Name the structure labelled 58.
59.	Name the structure labelled 59.
60.	Name the structure labelled 60.

MRI Head

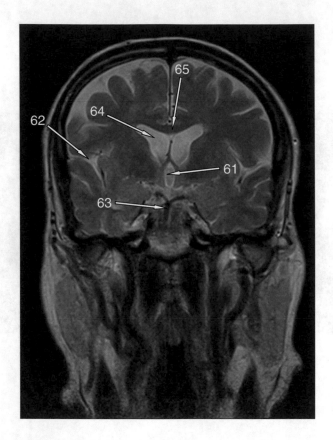

Questions	
61.	Name the structure labelled 61.
62.	Name the structure labelled 62.
63.	Name the structure labelled 63.
64.	Name the structure labelled 64.
65.	Name the structure labelled 65.

MRA

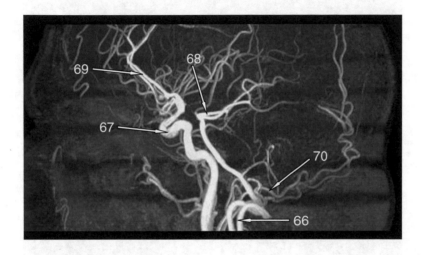

Questions	
66.	Name the structure labelled 66.
67.	Name the structure labelled 67.
68.	Name the structure labelled 68.
69.	Name the structure labelled 69.
70.	Name the structure labelled 70.

CT Abdomen

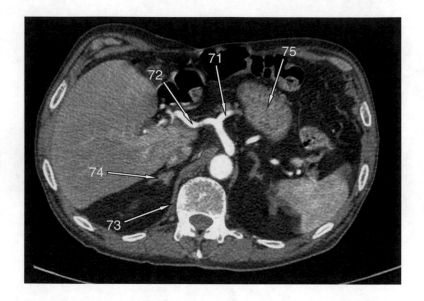

Questions	
71.	Name the structure labelled 71.
72.	Name the structure labelled 72.
73.	Name the structure labelled 73.
74.	Name the structure labelled 74.
75.	Name the structure labelled 75.

Lumbar Spine Radiograph

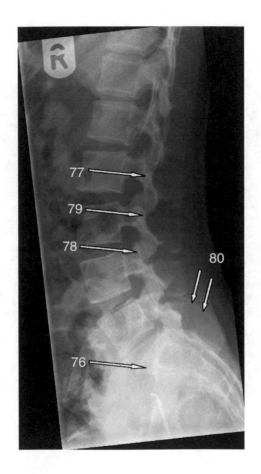

Questions	
76.	Name the structure labelled 76.
77.	Name the structure labelled 77.
78.	Name the structure labelled 78.
79.	Name the structure labelled 79.
80.	Name the structure labelled 80.

Hysterosalpingogram (HSG)

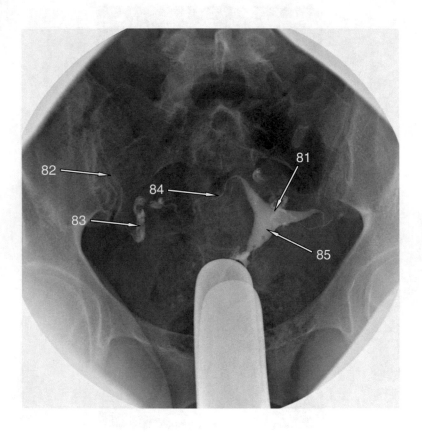

Questions	
81.	Name the structure labelled 81.
82.	Name the structure labelled 82.
83.	Name the structure labelled 83.
84.	Name the structure labelled 84.
85.	Name the structure labelled 85.

DSA

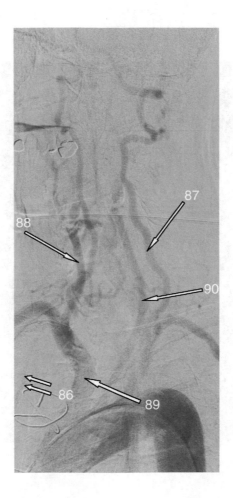

Questions	
86.	Name the structure labelled 86.
87.	Name the structure labelled 87.
88.	Name the structure labelled 88.
89.	Name the structure labelled 89.
90.	Name the structure labelled 90.

MRI Pelvis

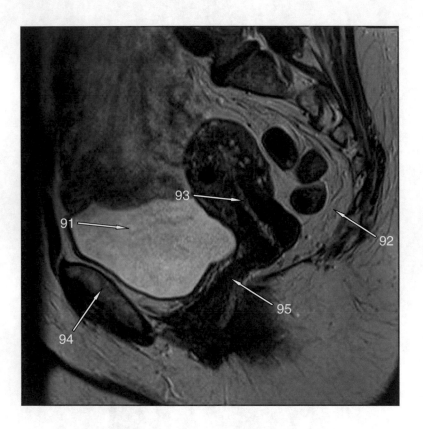

Questions	
91.	Name the structure labelled 91.
92.	Name the structure labelled 92.
93.	Name the structure labelled 93.
94.	Name the structure labelled 94.
95.	Name the structure labelled 95.

CT Abdomen

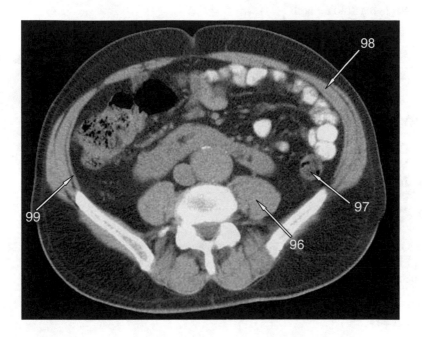

Questions

96.   Name the structure labelled 96.

97.   Name the structure labelled 97.

98.   Name the structure labelled 98.

99.   Name the structure labelled 99.

100. Name the anatomical variant seen in the image.

Test 6 Answers

Cervical Spine Radiograph

1. Head of left clavicle
2. Right first rib
3. Left transverse process of T1
4. Right mastoid air cells
5. Left angle of mandible

C7 vertebra is found as it has downward-pointing transverse processes, unlike the thoracic vertebrae, which have upward pointing transverse processes.

DSA

6. Confluence of venous sinuses (torcula herophili)
7. Vein of Labbe
8. Internal cerebral vein
9. Sigmoid sinus
10. Cavernous sinus

This is a digitally subtracted cerebral angiogram in the venous phase. Torcula herophili is the confluence of the sinuses and turns to one side (usually to the left side) to become the transverse sinus.

MRI Head

11. Quadrigeminal cistern
12. Basilar artery
13. Cerebellar folia
14. Optic chiasm
15. Left internal carotid artery

MRI Pelvis

16. Symphysis pubis
17. Ischioanal (rectal) fossa
18. Prostate (peripheral zone)
19. Left pectineus muscle
20. Left spermatic cord

The prostate is divided into three anatomical zones: transitional, central and peripheral zones. However on T2-weighted MR images only two zones can be distinguished: the peripheral and central zones. The majority of prostate cancers occur in the peripheral zone.

MRI Chest

21. Fundus of stomach
22. Right subclavian vein
23. Pulmonary trunk
24. Gallbladder
25. Right atrium

CT Heart

26. Left upper lobe bronchus
27. Descending thoracic aorta
28. Left coronary artery
29. Right superior pulmonary artery
30. Right coronary artery

The pericardium can be identified as a thin dense line separated from the myocardium by a thin layer of epicardial fat. Coronary artery dominance is determined by the vessel that supplies the inferior and lateral walls of the left ventricle.

DSA

31. Anterior cusp of aortic valve
32. Left posterior cusp of aortic valve
33. Circumflex artery
34. Right coronary artery
35. Left subclavian artery

The ascending aorta begins at the aortic valve at the level of the lower border of the third costal cartilage. There are three cusps of the aortic valve of which two are related to the respective sinuses that give rise to coronary arteries.

Ultrasound Abdomen

36. Middle hepatic vein
37. Inferior vena cava
38. Segment 8 of the liver
39. Right dome of diaphragm
40. Segment 4 of the liver

The hepatic veins divide the liver vertically and portal veins divide the liver horizontally into segments. These are named using the Couinaud classification. The hepatic veins can therefore be used to identify liver segments and allow a precise description of the position of focal lesions.

Barium Enema

41. Transverse colon
42. Right anterior superior iliac spine
43. Ascending colon
44. Sigmoid colon
45. Left obturator foramen

CT Head

46. Left foramen ovale
47. Left foramen spinosum
48. Right caroticojugular spine
49. Nasal septum
50. Right pterygoid (vidian) canal

The pterygoid canal (also vidian canal) is a passage in the skull leading from just anterior to the foramen lacerum in the middle cranial fossa to the pterygopalatine fossa. It transmits the nerve of the pterygoid canal and its corresponding artery. It is an important landmark in transnasal endoscopic surgery for identifying the petrous part of the internal carotid artery.

Ultrasound Abdomen

51. Inferior vena cava
52. Left rectus abdominis muscle
53. Left lobe of liver
54. Uncinate process/head of pancreas
55. Common bile duct

The pancreas lies at L1.

The dorsal aspect of the head takes the shape of a hook surrounding the right side of the superior mesenteric vein; the sharp left-pointing tip of the hook behind the vein forms the uncinate process. The splenic vein runs from the left along the dorsal border of the tail and body to the superior mesenteric vein, where these veins join to form the portal vein behind the 'neck' of the pancreas.

The uncinate process is the only part of the pancreas to lie posterior to the superior mesenteric vessels.

The pancreas tends to be hyperechoic and pancreatic malignancies are hypoechoic.

CT Chest

56. Trachea
57. Right lobe of thyroid gland
58. Left internal jugular vein
59. Oesophagus
60. Left subscapularis muscle

MRI Head

61. Third ventricle
62. Right Sylvian fissure
63. Basilar artery
64. Right lateral ventricle (body of)
65. Body of corpus callosum

The Sylvian fissure divides the frontal and parietal lobe above from the temporal lobe below. It appears around the 14th week of gestation and is one the most prominent fissures of the brain. The M1 segment of the middle cerebral artery lies within this fissure.

MRA

66. Vertebral artery
67. Internal carotid artery (cavernous portion)
68. Posterior cerebral artery
69. Anterior cerebral artery
70. Posterior inferior cerebellar artery

The intracranial carotid artery has a very tortuous course; this may have a role in reducing the pulsating force to the brain. Its intracranial course has been divided into seven anatomical segments according to Bouthillier's classification.

CT Abdomen

71. Splenic artery
72. Common hepatic artery
73. Right crus of diaphragm
74. Right adrenal gland
75. Stomach

The coeliac artery arises ventrally from the abdominal aorta at T12. This image depicts the 'seagull sign' with the ceoliac trunk dividing into the splenic and hepatic arteries. The left gastric artery isn't demonstrated in this plane.

Also note that the suprarenal glands have a linear 'V' (right) or a triangular or 'Y' shape (left).

The right adrenal gland lies posterior to the IVC, medial to the right lobe of the liver and lateral to the right diaphragmatic crus.

Lumbar Spine Radiograph

76. Sacral promontory
77. Transverse process of L3 vertebra
78. Superior articular process of L4 vertebra
79. Inferior articular process (facet) of L2 vertebra
80. Iliac crest

Use the L5 vertebral body as a landmark for identifying the correct level of the lumbar vertebra and hence its respective parts. Oblique views of the lumbar spine are used to see the intervertebral foramina and the pars interarticularis (Scotty dog sign).

Hysterosalpingogram (HSG)

81. Uterine fundus
82. Right sacroiliac joint
83. Ampulla of right uterine tube
84. Isthmus of right uterine tube
85. Body of uterus

DSA

86. Right internal thoracic artery
87. Left vertebral artery
88. Right common carotid artery
89. Brachiocephalic artery
90. Left common carotid artery

The normal patterns of the branches of the aorta are seen in only 65 % of subjects. The vertebral artery arises from the first part of the subclavian artery. The left vertebral artery is dominant in 80 % of cases.

MRI Pelvis

91. Bladder
92. Mesorectum
93. Endometrium
94. Pubic symphysis
95. Vagina

The MR appearance of normal endometrium is best demonstrated on T2-weighted images because the uterus has homogeneous intermediate signal intensity with T1-weighted sequences. T2-weighted images delineate the uterine zonal anatomy. The normal endometrium is of uniformly high signal intensity, and the inner myometrium, or junctional zone, is of uniformly low signal intensity.

CT Abdomen

96. Left psoas major muscle
97. Descending colon
98. Right internal oblique muscle
99. Right transversus abdominis muscle
100. Horseshoe kidney

Horseshoe kidney is a congenital anomaly affecting about 1 in 400 people. The central portion of the kidney is found below the inferior mesenteric artery.

Test 7

7

(You have 90 minutes to complete 100 questions)

P. Borg et al., *Radiological Anatomy for FRCR Part 1*,
DOI 10.1007/978-3-642-41166-3_7, © Springer-Verlag Berlin Heidelberg 2014

Foot Radiograph

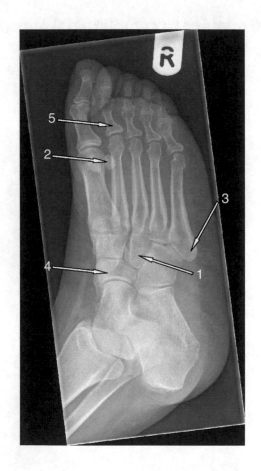

Questions	
1.	Name the structure labelled 1.
2.	Name the structure labelled 2.
3.	Name the structure labelled 3.
4.	Name the structure labelled 4.
5.	Name the structure labelled 5.

MRA

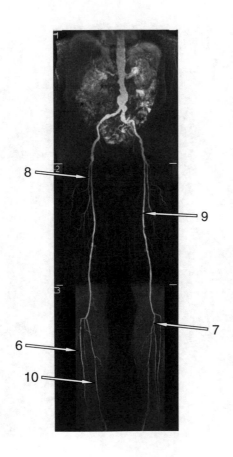

Questions	
6.	Name the structure labelled 6.
7.	Name the structure labelled 7.
8.	Name the structure labelled 8.
9.	Name the structure labelled 9.
10.	Name the structure labelled 10.

Cervical Spine Radiograph

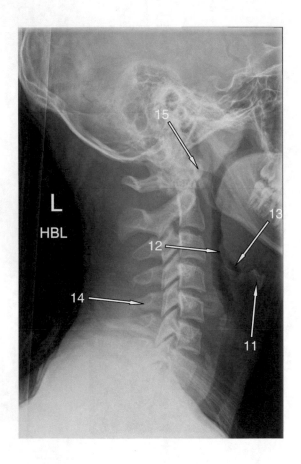

Questions	
11.	Name the structure labelled 11.
12.	Name the structure labelled 12.
13.	Name the structure labelled 13.
14.	Name the structure labelled 14.
15.	Name the structure labelled 15.

CT Abdomen

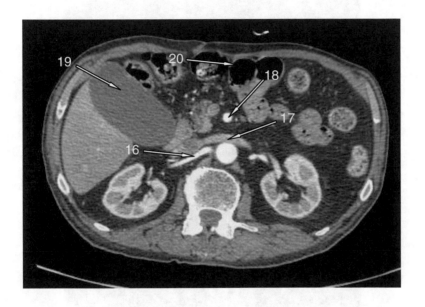

Questions	
16.	Name the structure labelled 16.
17.	Name the structure labelled 17.
18.	Name the structure labelled 18.
19.	Name the structure labelled 19.
20.	Name the structure labelled 20.

MRI Head

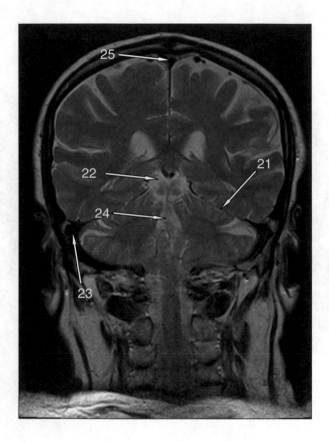

Questions	
21.	Name the structure labelled 21.
22.	Name the structure labelled 22.
23.	Name the structure labelled 23.
24.	Name the structure labelled 24.
25.	Name the structure labelled 25.

CT Chest

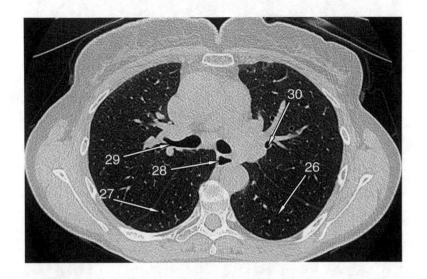

Questions	
26.	Name the structure labelled 26.
27.	Name the structure labelled 27.
28.	Name the structure labelled 28.
29.	Name the structure labelled 29.
30.	Name the structure labelled 30.

CT Pelvis

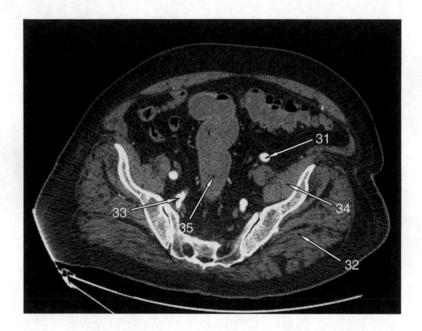

Questions	
31.	Name the structure labelled 31.
32.	Name the structure labelled 32.
33.	Name the structure labelled 33.
34.	Name the structure labelled 34.
35.	Name the structure labelled 35.

Chest Radiograph

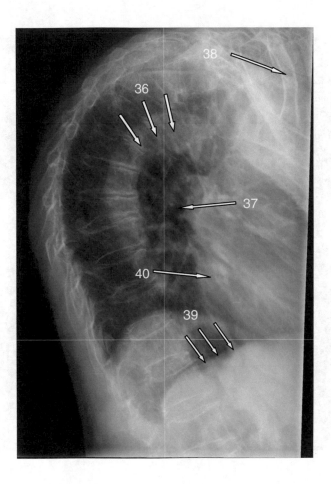

Questions	
36.	Name the structure labelled 36.
37.	Name the hilar structure labelled 37.
38.	Name the hilar structure labelled 38.
39.	Name the structure labelled 39.
40.	Name the heart chamber labelled 40.

CT Head

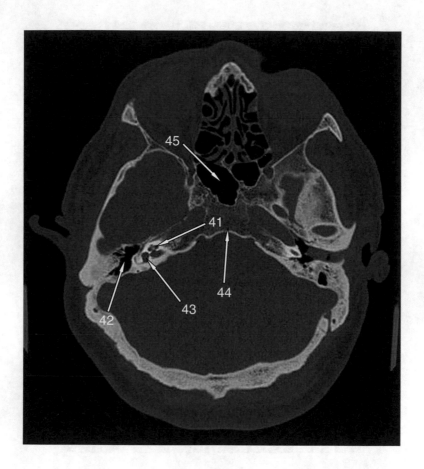

Questions	
41.	Name the structure labelled 41.
42.	Name the structure labelled 42.
43.	Name the structure labelled 43.
44.	Name the structure labelled 44.
45.	Name the structure labelled 45.

DSA

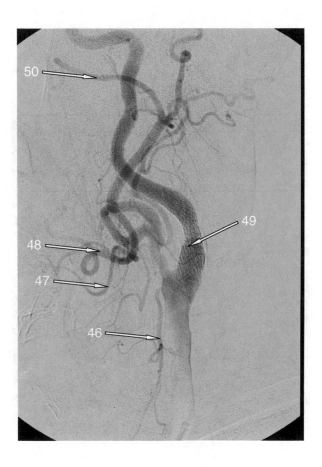

Questions	
46.	Name the structure labelled 46.
47.	Name the structure labelled 47.
48.	Name the structure labelled 48.
49.	Name the structure labelled 49.
50.	Name the structure labelled 50.

Knee Radiograph

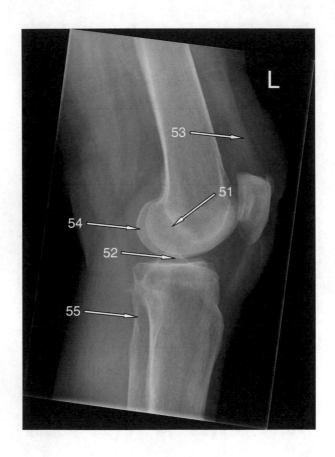

Questions	
51.	Name the structure labelled 51.
52.	Name the structure labelled 52.
53.	Name the structure labelled 53.
54.	Name the structure labelled 54.
55.	Name the structure labelled 55.

Barium Swallow (Anterior View Neck)

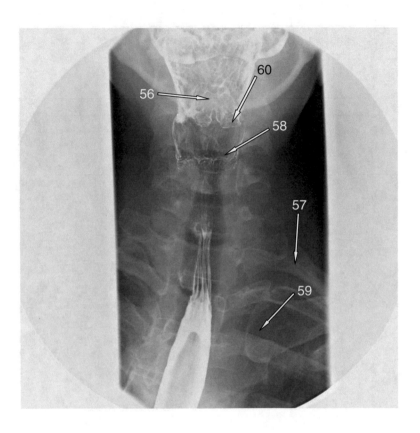

Questions	
56.	Name the structure labelled 56.
57.	Name the structure labelled 57.
58.	Name the structure labelled 58.
59.	Name the structure labelled 59.
60.	Name the structure labelled 60.

Chest Radiograph

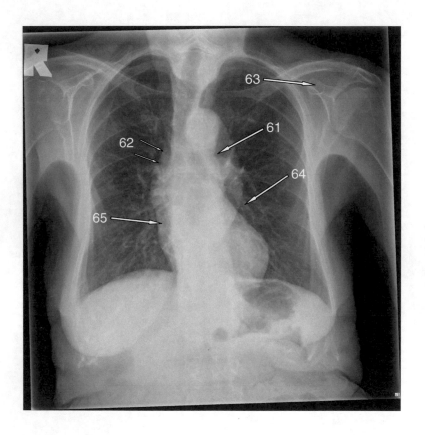

Questions	
61.	Name the structure labelled 61.
62.	Name the structure labelled 62.
63.	Name the structure labelled 63.
64.	Name the structure labelled 64.
65.	Name the structure labelled 65.

MRI Pelvis

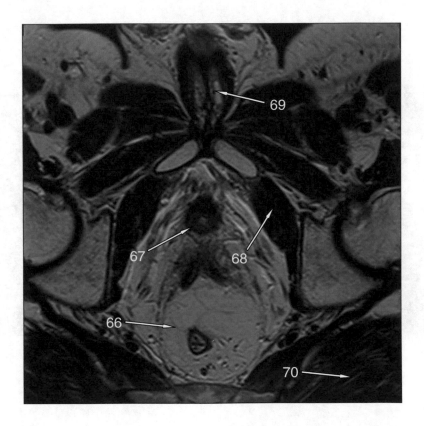

Questions	
66.	Name the structure labelled 66.
67.	Name the structure labelled 67.
68.	Name the structure labelled 68.
69.	Name the structure labelled 69.
70.	Name the structure labelled 70.

CT Neck

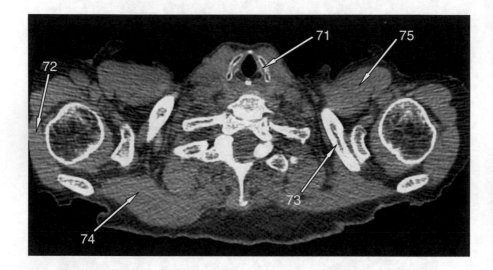

Questions	
71.	Name the structure labelled 71.
72.	Name the structure labelled 72.
73.	Name the structure labelled 73.
74.	Name the structure labelled 74.
75.	Name the structure labelled 75.

CT Chest

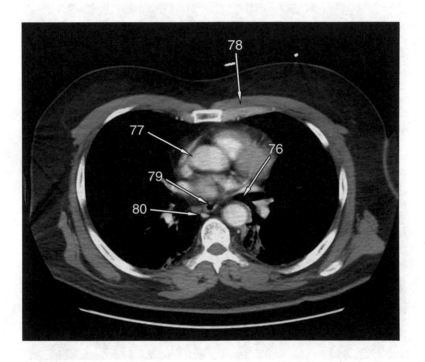

Questions	
76.	Name the structure labelled 76.
77.	Name the structure labelled 77.
78.	Name the structure labelled 78.
79.	Name the structure labelled 79.
80.	Name the structure labelled 80.

MRI Neck

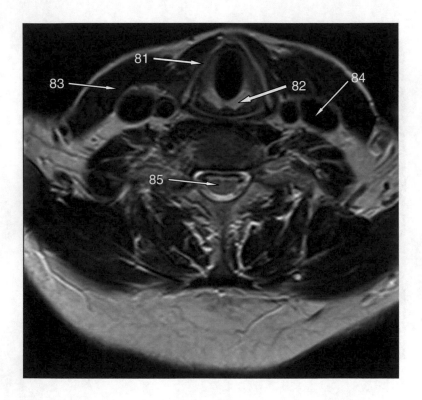

Questions	
81.	Name the structure labelled 81.
82.	Name the structure labelled 82.
83.	Name the structure labelled 83.
84.	Name the structure labelled 84.
85.	Name the structure labelled 85.

Wrist Radiograph

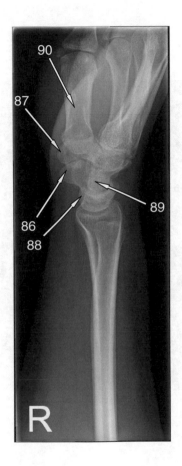

Questions	
86.	Name the structure labelled 86.
87.	Name the structure labelled 87.
88.	Name the structure labelled 88.
89.	Name the structure labelled 89.
90.	Name the structure labelled 90.

Abdominal Ultrasound

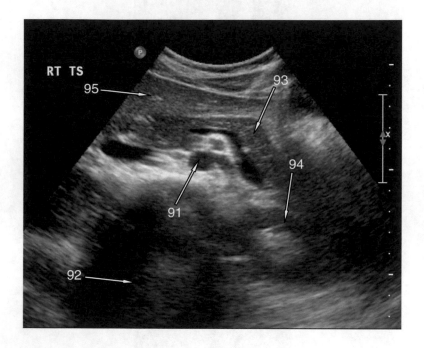

Questions	
91.	Name the structure labelled 91.
92.	Name the structure labelled 92.
93.	Name the structure labelled 93.
94.	Name the structure labelled 94.
95.	Name the structure labelled 95.

MRI Head

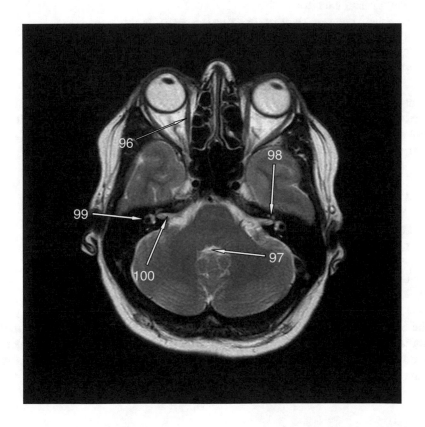

Questions	
96.	Name the structure labelled 96.
97.	Name the structure labelled 97.
98.	Name the structure labelled 98.
99.	Name the structure labelled 99.
100.	Name the structure labelled 100.

Test 7 Answers

Foot Radiograph

1. Right lateral cuneiform
2. Sesamoid bones in right flexor hallucis brevis muscle
3. Tuberosity of base of right 5th metatarsal
4. Right navicular
5. Proximal phalanx of right second toe

Some of the most common accessory ossicles in the foot are os trigonum, posterior to talus; os vesalianum, base of 5th metatarsal; os peroneum, between cuboid and base of 5th metatarsal within tendon of peroneus brevis muscle; and os tibiale externum, medial to tuberosity of navicular within tendon of tibialis posterior.

MRA

6. Right anterior tibial artery (AT)
7. Left tibioperoneal trunk (TPT)
8. Right profunda femoris artery (PFA)
9. Left superficial femoral artery (SFA)
10. Right posterior tibial artery (PTA)

The SFA has no significant branches in the thigh and has a vertical course in the thigh. Below the knee the popliteal artery divides into the tiobioperoneal trunk and anterior tibial artery over the proximal tibiofibular joint. The posterior tibial artery is the most medial vessel seen in the lower leg.

Cervical Spine Radiograph

11. Body of hyoid bone
12. Epiglottis
13. Vallecula
14. Spinous process of C5 vertebra
15. Anterior arch of C1 vertebra (Atlas)

CT Abdomen

16. Right renal artery
17. Left renal vein
18. Superior mesenteric artery
19. Gallbladder
20. Transverse colon

This is an arterial phase CT at L1/L2; the superior mesenteric vein lies to the left of its corresponding artery. The renal medullary pyramids are seen in their full length at the level of the hilum. The gastroduodenal artery is visible just lateral to the pancreas in this image.

MRI Head

21. Tentorium cerebelli (Left)
22. Quadrigeminal cistern
23. Right sigmoid sinus
24. Fourth ventricle
25. Superior sagittal sinus

CT Chest

26. Left lower lobe (Superior/apical segment of)
27. Right lower lobe
28. Oesophagus
29. Bronchus intermedius
30. Left superior lobe bronchus

CT Pelvis

31. Left external iliac artery
32. Left gluteus maximus muscle
33. Right internal iliac artery
34. Left iliacus muscle
35. Rectum

This is a CT angiogram axial view showing the division of the right internal iliac artery into its anterior and posterior trunk. The internal iliac artery arises in front of the sacroiliac joint at the level of L5/S1. Remember that the aorta normally bifurcates at the level of L4.

Chest Radiograph

36. Arch of aorta
37. Left main bronchus
38. Clavicle
39. Right dome of diaphragm
40. Left atrium

Lateral chest x-ray demonstrating kyphosis. Remember that the left main bronchus, being more horizontal, is seen as a circular structure. The left pulmonary artery is comma-shaped as it arches over the left main bronchus.

The following points help identify the domes of the diaphragm:
• Air within the gastric fundus lies under the left dome.
• The heart shadow obscures part of the left dome.
• The inferior vena cava may be seen traversing the right dome.

CT Head

41. Right cochlea
42. Right mastoid antrum
43. Right vestibule
44. Clivus
45. Sphenoidal sinus

The spiral cochlea is demonstrated in this axial CT on bone window settings. Therefore the cerebellar hemispheres, temporal lobe and the soft tissues of the galea are barely identifiable. The bony labyrinth consists of a vestibule, which communicates posteriorly with the semicircular canals (of which there are three: superior, lateral and posterior) and anteriorly with the spiral cochlea.

DSA

46. Superior thyroid artery
47. Lingual artery
48. Facial artery
49. Internal carotid artery
50. Maxillary artery

A useful mnemonic for memorising the branches of the external carotid artery (inferior to superior) is '*S*ome *A*natomists *L*ike *F*reaking *O*ut *M*edical *S*tudents'.

- Superior thyroid artery
- Ascending pharyngeal artery
- Lingual artery
- Facial artery
- Occipital artery
- Maxillary artery
- Superficial temporal artery

Knee Radiograph

51. Intercondylar fossa (Left)
52. Tubercles of intercondylar eminence/tibial spine (Left)
53. Left quadriceps tendon
54. Left femoral condyle
55. Neck of fibula (Left)

Barium Swallow (Anterior View Neck)

56. Epiglottis
57. Left first rib
58. Piriform fossa
59. Medial end of left clavicle
60. Valleculae

In the upper part of this image, the en face view of the base of the tongue is seen. The median glossoepiglottic fold crosses from tongue base to epiglottis, dividing the retroglottic space into two cup-shaped valleculae (60).

Chest Radiograph

61. Aortopulmonary window
62. SVC
63. Left coracoid process
64. Left inferior pulmonary artery
65. Right atrium

MRI Pelvis

66. Mesorectal fat
67. Prostate
68. Left obturator internus
69. Corpus cavernosum (left)
70. Left gluteus maximus muscle

CT Neck

71. Thyroid cartilage
72. Right deltoid
73. Left clavicle
74. Right trapezius muscle
75. Left pectoralis major muscle

This axial CT is taken with the arms raised above the head.

CT Chest

76. Left main bronchus
77. Ascending thoracic aorta
78. Left pectoralis major muscle
79. Oesophagus
80. Azygos vein

Note the hemiazygos vein behind the descending thoracic aorta.
The azygos vein drains the posterior walls of the thorax and abdomen into the superior vena cava at T4.

MRI Neck

81. Thyroid cartilage
82. Arytenoid cartilage
83. Right sternocleidomastoid muscle
84. Left internal jugular vein
85. Spinal cord

This is an axial T2-weighted MRI at the level of the glottis ldemonstrating a complete ring of cartilage. The thyroid cartilage is triangular on axial section with the apex pointing anteriorly with the cricoid cartilage seen posterior to the arytenoid cartilage. The paralaryngeal space is between the larynx and thyroid cartilage and is an important landmark in the staging of laryngeal tumours.

Wrist Radiograph

86. Right scaphoid
87. Right pisiform
88. Right lunate
89. Right capitate
90. Right thumb metacarpal

The lateral wrist X-ray is useful in determining lunate dislocation. Always look at the alignment of the lunate and capitate in these films. Failure to diagnose this disorder can result in permanent impairment of the median nerve if it is compressed by the lunate.

Abdominal Ultrasound

91. Abdominal aorta
92. Lumbar vertebra
93. Pancreas
94. Left renal cortex
95. Left lobe of liver

MRI Head

96. Right medial rectus muscle
97. Fourth ventricle
98. Left cochlea
99. Right semicircular canal
100. Right vestibulocochlear nerve in internal acoustic canal

This is an axial T2 MRI showing the internal auditory meatus at the level of the VIII (vestibulocochlear) nerve. The extraocular muscles are also demonstrated. Fat saturation sequences are used to help distinguish the optic nerve and its sleeve of dura and CSF from the surrounding fat.

Test 8

8

(You have 90 minutes to complete 100 questions)

P. Borg et al., *Radiological Anatomy for FRCR Part 1*,
DOI 10.1007/978-3-642-41166-3_8, © Springer-Verlag Berlin Heidelberg 2014

DSA

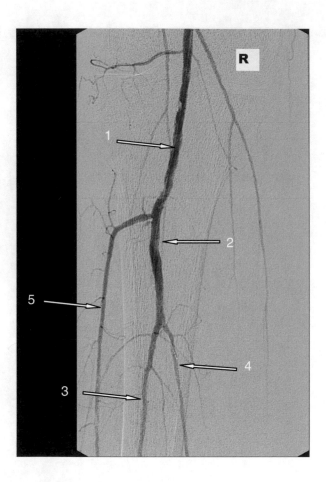

Questions	
1.	Name the structure labelled 1.
2.	Name the structure labelled 2.
3.	Name the structure labelled 3.
4.	Name the structure labelled 4.
5.	Name the structure labelled 5.

CT Head

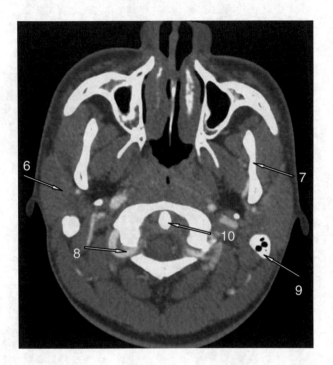

Shoulder Radiograph

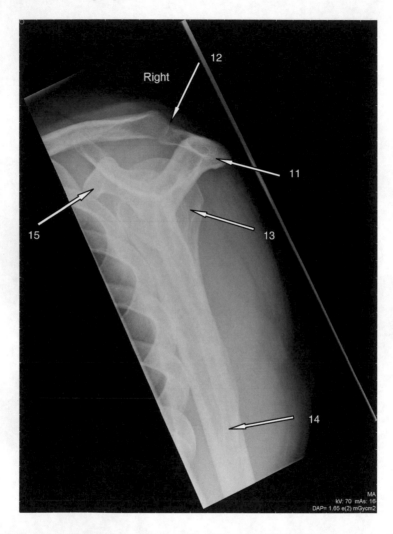

Questions	
11.	Name the structure labelled 11.
12.	Name the structure labelled 12.
13.	Name the structure labelled 13.
14.	Name the structure labelled 14.
15.	Name the structure labelled 15.

CT Abdomen

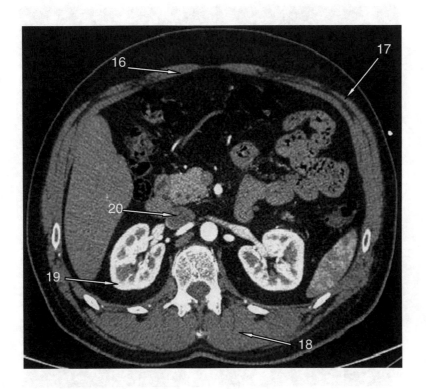

Questions	
16.	Name the structure labelled 16.
17.	Name the structure labelled 17.
18.	Name the structure labelled 18.
19.	Name the structure labelled 19.
20.	Name the structure labelled 20.

MRI Head

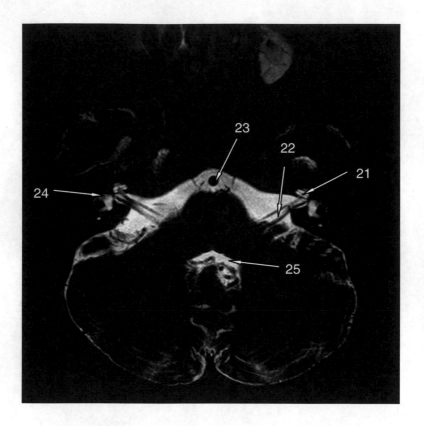

Questions	
21.	Name the structure labelled 21.
22.	Name the structure labelled 22.
23.	Name the structure labelled 23.
24.	Name the structure labelled 24.
25.	Name the structure labelled 25.

Foot Radiograph

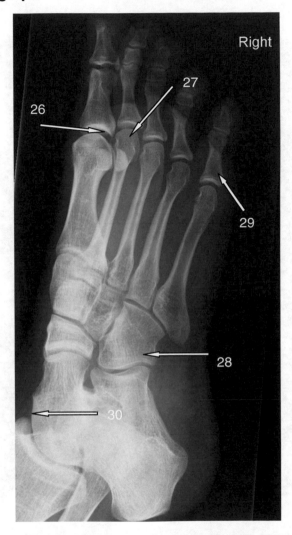

Questions	
26.	Name the structure labelled 26.
27.	Name the structure labelled 27.
28.	Name the structure labelled 28.
29.	Name the structure labelled 29.
30.	Name the structure labelled 30.

MRI Spine

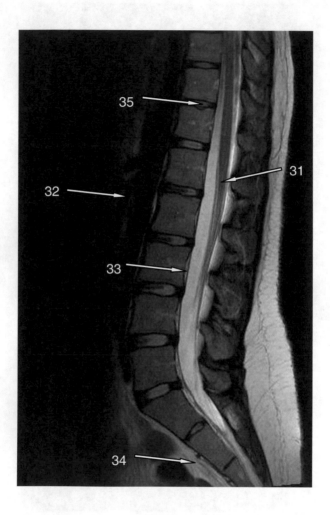

Questions	
31.	Name the structure labelled 31.
32.	Name the structure labelled 32.
33.	Name the structure labelled 33.
34.	Name the structure labelled 34.
35.	Name the structure labelled 35.

CT Heart

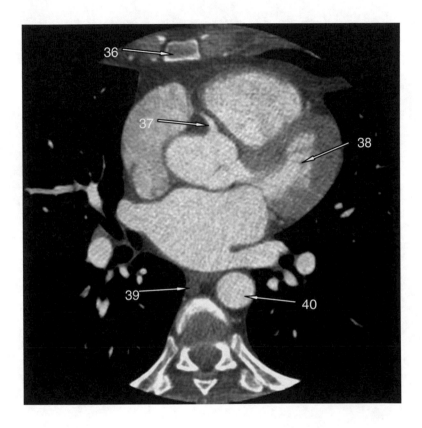

Questions	
36.	Name the structure labelled 36.
37.	Name the structure labelled 37.
38.	Name the structure labelled 38.
39.	Name the structure labelled 39.
40.	Name the structure labelled 40.

Abdominal Radiograph

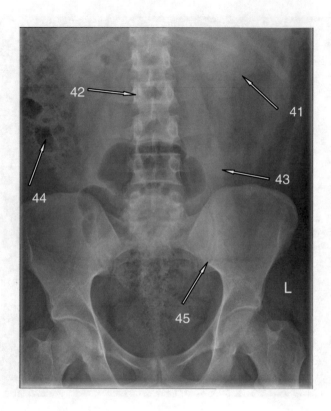

Questions	
41.	Name the structure labelled 41.
42.	Name the structure labelled 42.
43.	Name the structure labelled 43.
44.	Name the structure labelled 44.
45.	Name the structure labelled 45.

MRI PELVIS

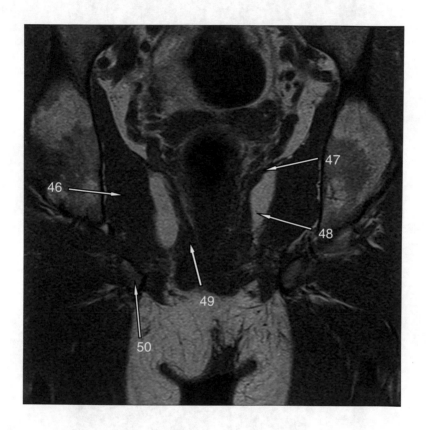

Questions	
46.	Name the structure labelled 46.
47.	Name the structure labelled 47.
48.	Name the structure labelled 48.
49.	Name the structure labelled 49.
50.	Name the structure labelled 50.

Skull Radiograph

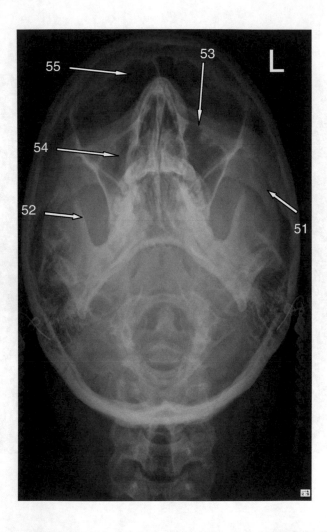

Questions	
51.	Name the structure labelled 51.
52.	Name the structure labelled 52.
53.	Name the structure labelled 53.
54.	Name the structure labelled 54.
55.	Name the structure labelled 55.

MRI Head

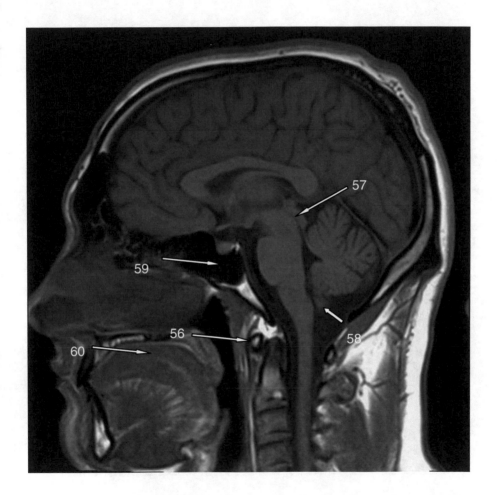

Questions	
56.	Name the structure labelled 56.
57.	Name the structure labelled 57.
58.	Name the structure labelled 58.
59.	Name the structure labelled 59.
60.	Name the structure labelled 60.

IVU

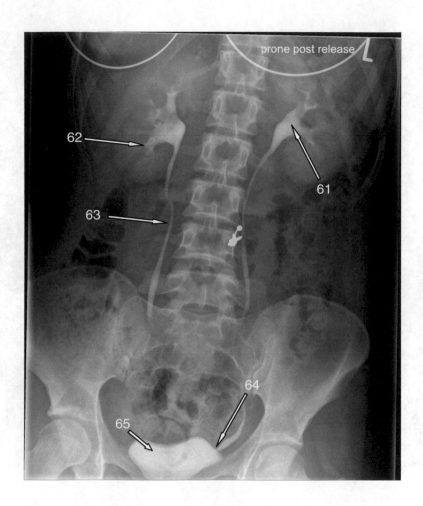

prone post release

62

61

63

64

65

Questions	
61.	Name the structure labelled 61.
62.	Name the structure labelled 62.
63.	Name the structure labelled 63.
64.	Name the structure labelled 64.
65.	Name the structure labelled 65.

Pelvic Radiograph

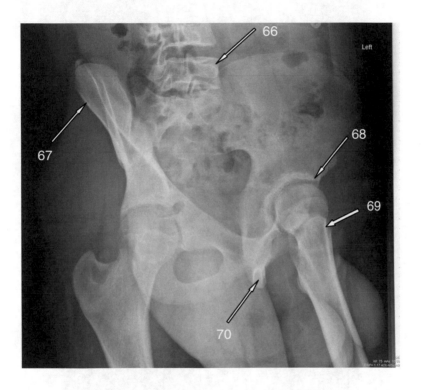

Questions	
66.	Name the structure labelled 66.
67.	Name the structure labelled 67.
68.	Name the structure labelled 68.
69.	Name the structure labelled 69.
70.	Name the structure labelled 70.

Knee Radiograph

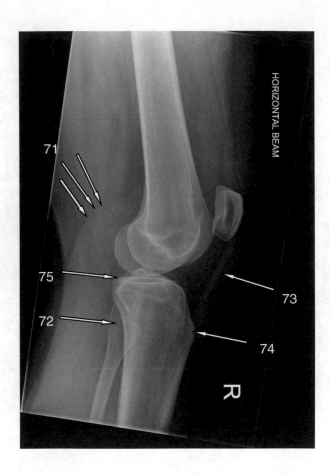

Questions	
71.	Name the structure labelled 71.
72.	Name the structure labelled 72.
73.	Name the structure labelled 73.
74.	Name the structure labelled 74.
75.	Name the structure labelled 75.

MRI Chest

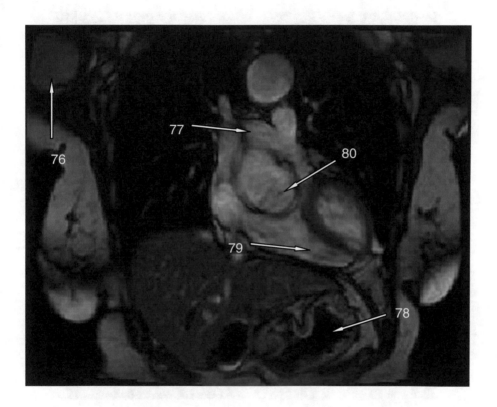

Questions	
76.	Name the structure labelled 76.
77.	Name the structure labelled 77.
78.	Name the structure labelled 78.
79.	Name the structure labelled 79.
80.	Name the structure labelled 80.

Cervical Spine Radiograph

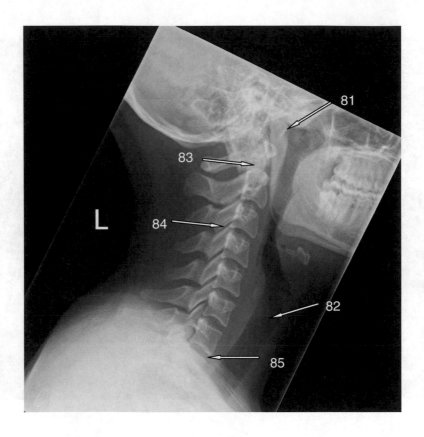

Questions
81. Name the structure labelled 81.
82. Name the structure labelled 82.
83. Name the structure labelled 83.
84. Name the structure labelled 84.
85. Name the structure labelled 85.

Mammogram

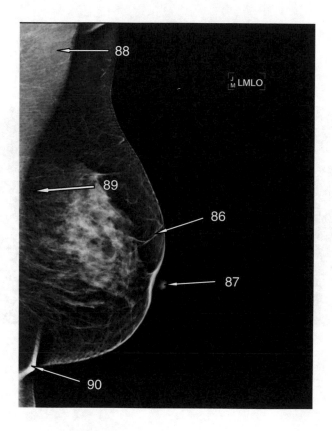

Questions	
86.	Name the structure labelled 86.
87.	Name the structure labelled 87.
88.	Name the structure labelled 88.
89.	Name the structure labelled 89.
90.	Name the structure labelled 90.

Orthopantomogram

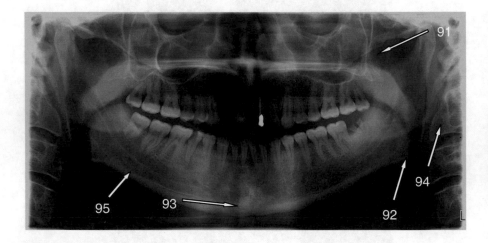

Questions	
91.	Name the structure labelled 91.
92.	Name the structure labelled 92.
93.	Name the structure labelled 93.
94.	Name the structure labelled 94.
95.	Name the structure labelled 95.

MRA

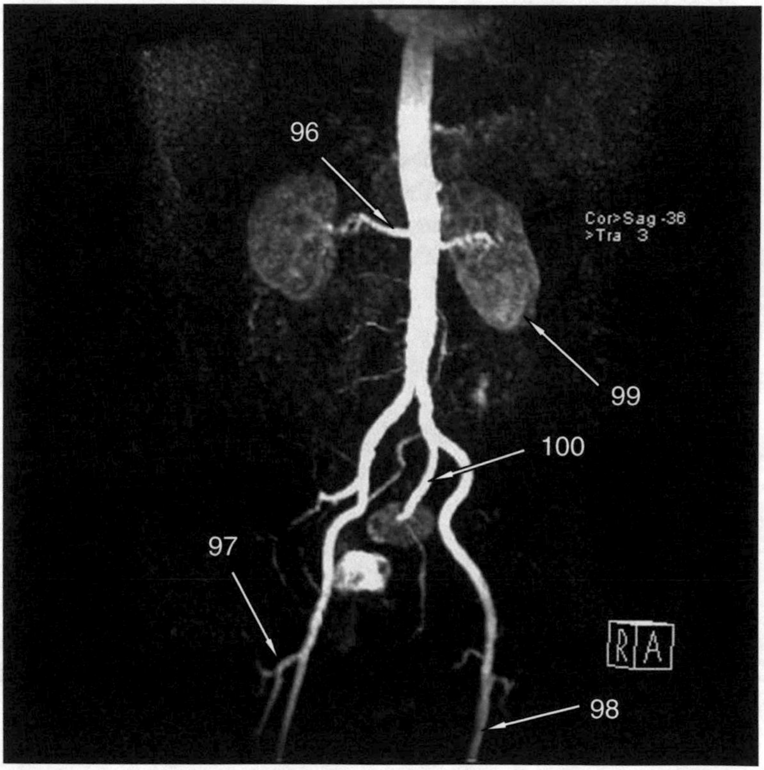

Questions	
96.	Name the structure labelled 96.
97.	Name the structure labelled 97.
98.	Name the structure labelled 98.
99.	Name the structure labelled 99.
100.	Name the structure labelled 100.

Test 8 Answers

DSA

1. Right popliteal artery
2. Right tibioperoneal trunk
3. Right peroneal artery
4. Right posterior tibial artery
5. Right anterior tibial artery

The superficial femoral artery continues as the popliteal artery, which in turn divides into major branches of the leg below the knee joint. Usually the anterior tibial artery comes off the lateral aspect of popliteal artery. It is common practice to palpate the posterior tibial arterial pulse posterior to the medial malleolus, which should help in remembering the medial most branch as posterior tibial artery.

CT Head

6. Right parotid gland
7. Left ramus of mandible
8. Right vertebral artery
9. Left mastoid process/air cells
10. Odontoid peg

The mastoids can be recognised by air cells (low attenuation areas in the bone). The parotid gland has superficial and deep parts and wraps around the ramus of mandible posteriorly.

Shoulder Radiograph

11. Right acromion process
12. Right acromioclavicular joint
13. Right glenoid
14. Right shaft of humerus
15. Right coracoid process

In case of fixed bony landmarks, it is important to recognise either the anterior or posterior most structure and work out the other parts of the scapula. On the Y view, the coracoid process is the anterior structure and closest to the ribs.

CT Abdomen

16. Right rectus abdominis muscle
17. Left external oblique muscle
18. Left erector spinae muscle
19. Right kidney (cortex)
20. Inferior vena cava

It is important to recognise the phase of contrast to correctly identify the vascular structures.

MRI Head

21. Left cochlea
22. Left vestibulocochlear (8th) nerve
23. Basilar artery
24. Right vestibular apparatus
25. Fourth ventricle

Foot Radiograph

26. Right 1st metatarsophalangeal joint
27. Right head of 2nd metatarsal
28. Right cuboid
29. Right proximal phalanx of little toe
30. Right talar dome/talus

Look carefully where the arrow head is indicated, i.e. joint or the bone. On an oblique view the 3rd metatarsal should be in line with the lateral cuneiform bone.

MRI Spine

31. Conus medullaris
32. Superior mesenteric artery
33. Posterior longitudinal ligament
34. Presacral fat
35. T11/12 intervertebral disc

The conus medullaris terminates at L1/L2 level. The presacral fat is high signal on T2-weighted image and blood vessels are of low signal intensity representing flow void. This image shows major blood vessel traversing the length of the abdomen, which can only be either abdominal aorta or IVC. Only the aorta gives off anterior branches. The coeliac artery and SMA are the two major anterior branches of abdominal aorta; hence 32 is a superior mesenteric artery.

CT Heart

36. Sternum
37. Right coronary artery
38. Left ventricle
39. Azygos vein
40. Descending aorta

On this view, recognising the anterior and posterior orientation is important in identifying the relevant anatomy. The right heart is anterior and closest to the sternum. The right coronary artery arises from the anterior (right) sinus of Valsalva of the aortic root and passes through the right atrioventricular groove anteriorly in the direction of sternum. In a normal heart, the left ventricular wall is more muscular than the right ventricle.

Abdominal Radiograph

41. Left kidney
42. Right pedicle of L2 vertebra
43. Left psoas muscle
44. Ascending colon
45. Left sacroiliac joint

MRI PELVIS

46. Right obturator internus muscle
47. Left levator ani muscle
48. Left ischioanal fossa
49. Right external anal sphincter
50. Right ischium

Skull Radiograph

51. Left zygomatic arch
52. Right coronoid process of mandible
53. Left orbital floor
54. Right maxillary sinus/antrum
55. Right frontal sinus

The zygomatic arch on this view looks like an elephant's trunk.

MRI Head

56. Anterior arch of atlas
57. Quadrigeminal plate
58. Cerebellar tonsil
59. Sphenoid sinus
60. Tongue

IVU

61. Left renal pelvis
62. Right inferior pole – minor calyx
63. Right ureter
64. Left vesicoureteric junction
65. Urinary bladder

Pelvic Radiograph

66. L5 vertebral body
67. Right ilium
68. Left acetabulum
69. Left neck of femur
70. Left ischial tuberosity

Knee Radiograph

71. Right gastrocnemius muscle
72. Right head of fibula
73. Right patellar ligament
74. Right tibial tuberosity
75. Right tibial plateau

MRI Chest

76. Right head of humerus
77. Right main pulmonary artery
78. Stomach
79. Right ventricle
80. Aortic root

On a coronal view, the right ventricle forms the base of the heart. The left ventricular wall is more muscular than the right. On this view, the pulmonary trunk can be seen originating from the right ventricle and dividing into right and left main pulmonary arteries.

Cervical Spine Radiograph

81. Mandibular condyle
82. Trachea
83. Dens
84. C3/C4 facet joint
85. C7/T1 intervertebral disc space

Mammogram

86. Cooper's ligament
87. Nipple
88. Pectoralis (major) muscle
89. Retroglandular fat
90. Inframammary skin fold

The MLO view is the pectoralis muscle should be convex anteriorly. Retroglandular fat can be seen as a lower density area between the pectoralis muscle and the anterior higher density glandular tissue of the breast anteriorly.

Orthopantomogram

91. Left coronoid process of mandible
92. Left angle of mandible
93. Symphysis menti
94. C2 vertebral body
95. Right body of mandible

MRA

96. Right renal artery
97. Right profunda femoris artery
98. Left superficial femoral artery
99. Left kidney
100. Left internal iliac artery

Test 9: Paediatrics

9

(You have 90 minutes to complete 100 questions)

Foot Radiograph

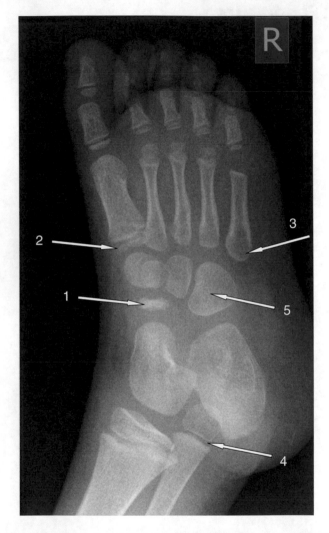

Questions	
1.	Name the structure labelled 1.
2.	Name the structure labelled 2.
3.	Name the muscle which attaches to the structure labelled 3.
4.	Name the structure labelled 4.
5.	Name the structure labelled 5.

Pelvic Radiograph

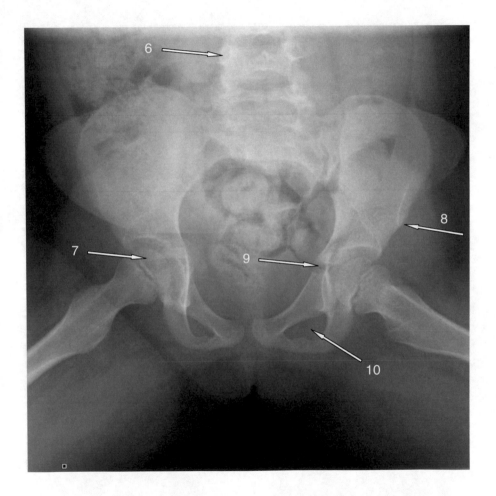

Questions	
6.	Name the structure labelled 6.
7.	Name the structure labelled 7.
8.	Name the muscle which attaches to the structure labelled 8.
9.	Name the structure labelled 9.
10.	Name the structure labelled 10.

CT Head

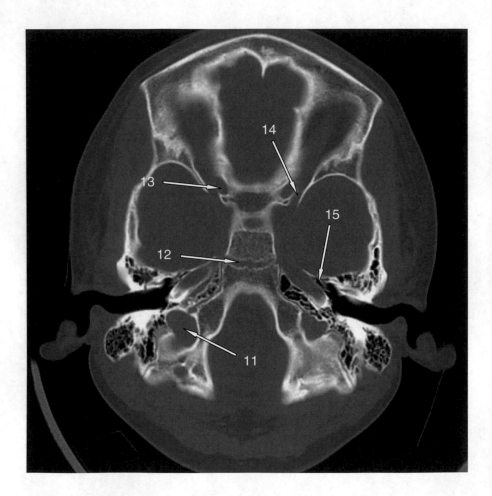

Questions	
11.	Name the structure labelled 11.
12.	Name the structure labelled 12.
13.	Name the structure labelled 13.
14.	Name the structure labelled 14.
15.	Name the air-filled structure labelled 15.

Lumbar Spine Radiograph

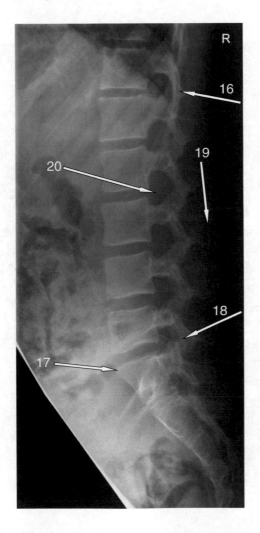

Questions	
16.	Name the structure labelled 16.
17.	Name the structure labelled 17.
18.	Name the structure labelled 18.
19.	Name the structure labelled 19.
20.	Which nerve passes through the structure labelled 20.

Elbow Radiograph

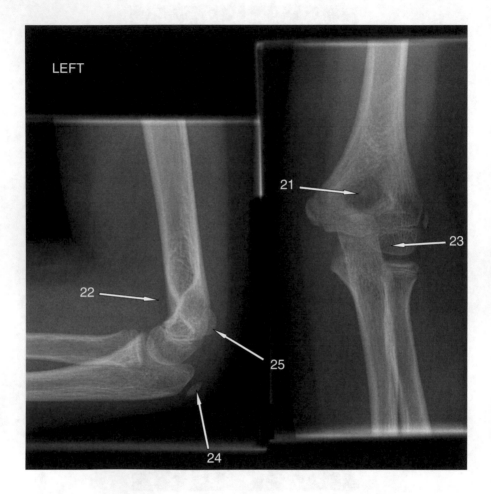

Questions	
21.	Name the structure labelled 21.
22.	Name the lucent triangular area labelled 22.
23.	Name the structure labelled 23.
24.	Name the structure labelled 24.
25.	Name the structure labelled 25.

MRI Head

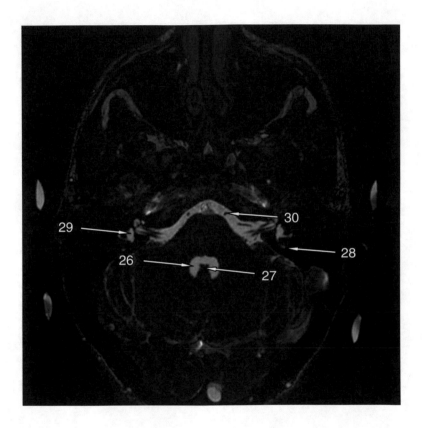

Questions	
26.	Name the structure labelled 26.
27.	Name the structure labelled 27.
28.	Name the structure labelled 28.
29.	Name the structure labelled 29.
30.	Name the structure labelled 30.

Barium Meal

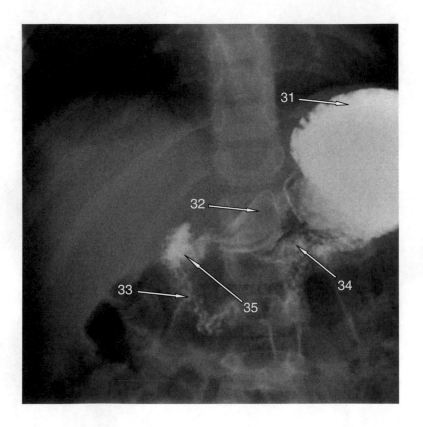

Questions	
31.	Name the structure labelled 31.
32.	Name the structure labelled 32.
33.	Name the structure labelled 33.
34.	Name the structure labelled 34.
35.	Name the structure labelled 35.

Neonatal Cranial Ultrasound

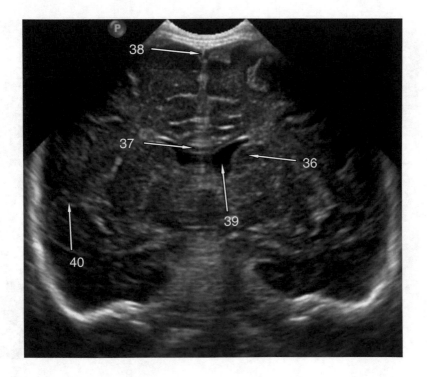

Questions	
36.	Name the structure labelled 36.
37.	Name the structure labelled 37.
38.	Name the structure labelled 38.
39.	Name the structure labelled 39.
40.	Name the structure labelled 40.

Shoulder Radiograph

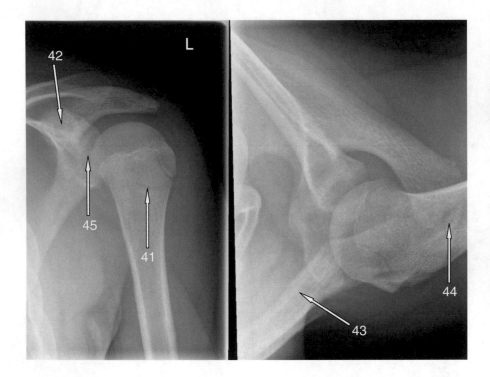

Questions	
41.	Name the structure labelled 41.
42.	Name the structure labelled 42.
43.	Name the structure labelled 43.
44.	Name the structure labelled 44, projected over the proximal humerus.
45.	Name the structure labelled 45.

Micturating Cystogram

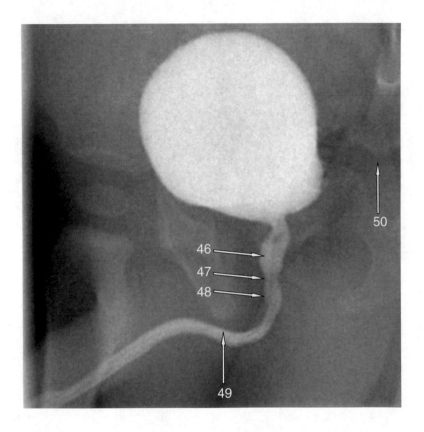

MRI Ankle

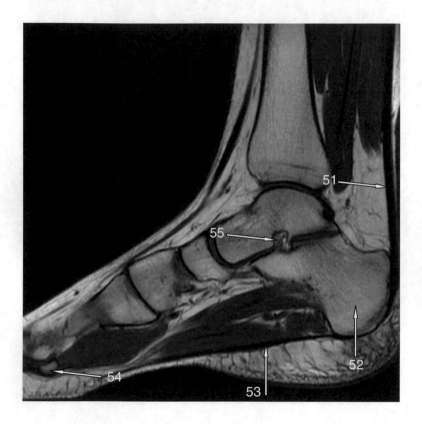

Questions	
51.	Name the structure labelled 51.
52.	Name the structure labelled 52.
53.	Name the structure labelled 53.
54.	Name the structure labelled 54.
55.	Name the structure labelled 55.

CT Temporal Bone

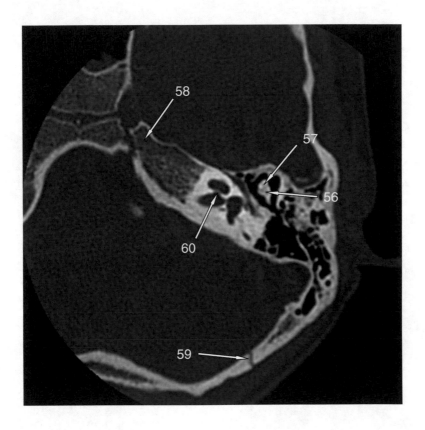

Questions	
56.	Name the structure labelled 56.
57.	Name the structure labelled 57.
58.	Name the structure labelled 58.
59.	Name the structure labelled 59.
60.	Name the structure labelled 60.

MRI Pelvis

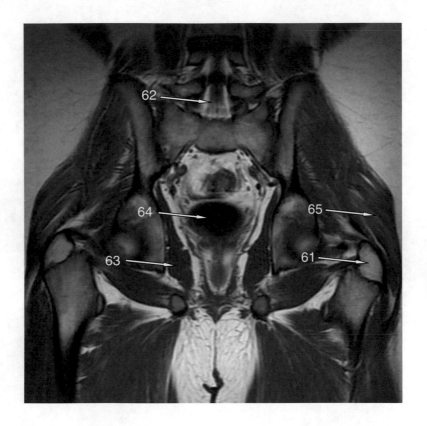

Questions	
61.	Name the structure labelled 61.
62.	Name the structure labelled 62.
63.	Name the structure labelled 63.
64.	Name the structure labelled 64.
65.	Name the structure labelled 65.

Chest Radiograph

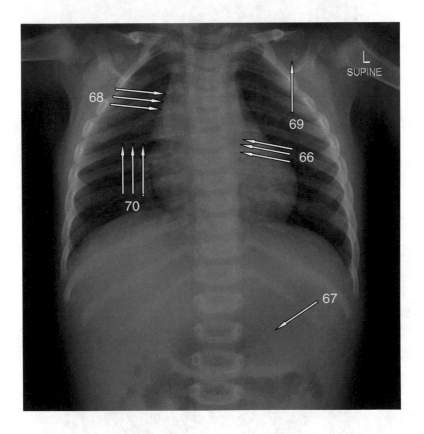

Questions	
66.	Name the structure labelled 66.
67.	Name the structure labelled 67.
68.	Name the structure labelled 68.
69.	Name the structure labelled 69.
70.	Name the structure labelled 70.

MRI Spine

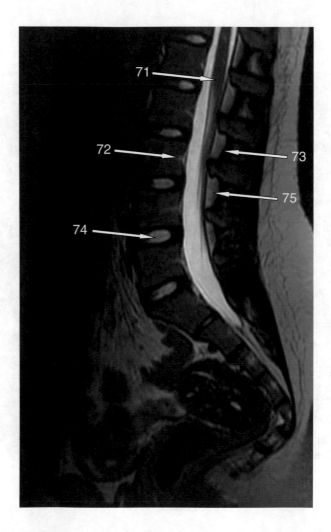

Questions	
71.	Name the structure labelled 71.
72.	Name the structure labelled 72.
73.	Name the structure labelled 73.
74.	Name the structure labelled 74.
75.	Name the structure labelled 75.

CT Chest

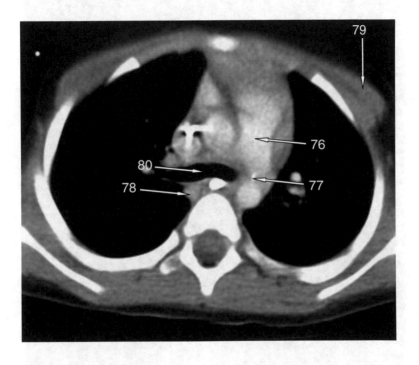

Questions	
76.	Name the structure labelled 76.
77.	Name the structure labelled 77.
78.	Name the structure labelled 78.
79.	Name the structure labelled 79.
80.	Name the structure labelled 80.

MRI Head

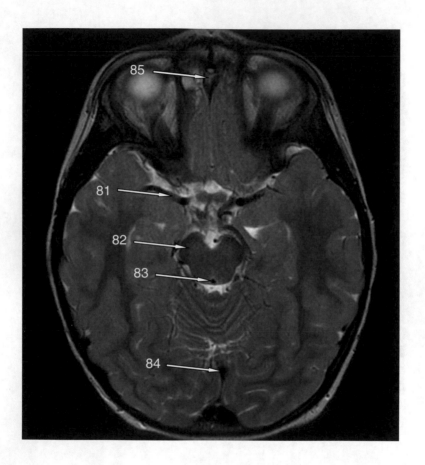

Questions	
81.	Name the structure labelled 81.
82.	Name the structure labelled 82.
83.	Name the structure labelled 83.
84.	Name the structure labelled 84.
85.	Name the structure labelled 85.

Ultrasound Hip

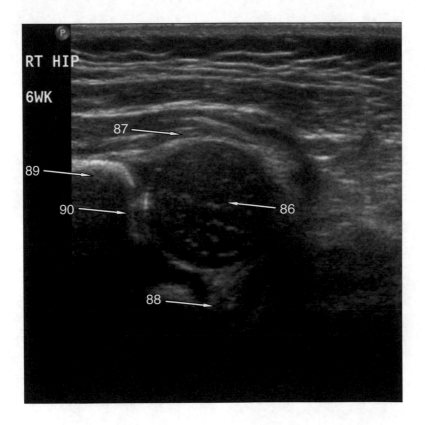

Questions	
86.	Name the structure labelled 86.
87.	Name the structure labelled 87.
88.	Name the structure labelled 88.
89.	Name the structure labelled 89.
90.	Name the structure labelled 90.

MRI Knee

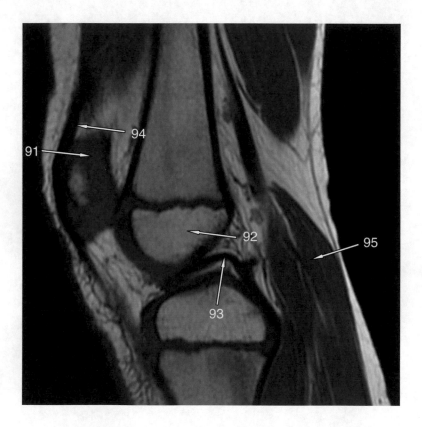

Questions	
91.	Name the structure labelled 91.
92.	Name the structure labelled 92.
93.	Name the structure labelled 93.
94.	Name the structure labelled 94.
95.	Name the structure labelled 95.

Ultrasound Abdomen

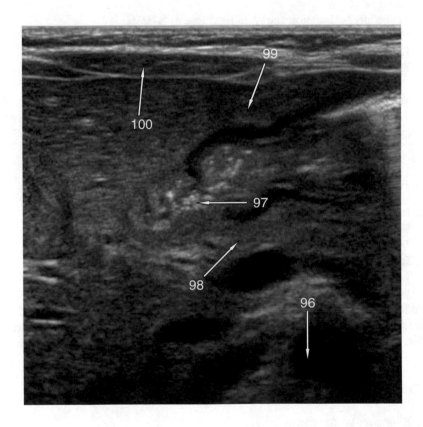

Questions	
96.	Name the structure labelled 96.
97.	Name the structure labelled 97.
98.	Name the structure labelled 98.
99.	Name the structure labelled 99.
100.	Name the structure labelled 100.

Test 9: Paediatric Answers

Foot Radiograph

1. Right navicular
2. Secondary ossification centre of right first metatarsal
3. Right peroneus brevis
4. Distal right fibular physis
5. Right cuboid

The navicular may appear irregular or fragmented as a normal variant during ossification. A residual cleft at the base of the first metatarsal following fusion of the secondary ossification centre is often mistaken for a fracture.

Pelvic Radiograph

6. Right pedicle of L4 vertebra
7. Right capital femoral epiphysis
8. Left rectus femoris – straight head
9. Left triradiate cartilage
10. Left obturator foramen

The frog lateral view is the best for assessment of slipped capital femoral epiphysis. Subtle signs of a slip include reduced height of the epiphysis and a widened growth plate.

CT Head

11. Right jugular foramen
12. Spheno-occipital or basi-occipital synchondrosis
13. Right optic canal
14. Left superior orbital fissure
15. Left Eustachian tube

The dural venous sinuses are often asymmetrical, with accompanying asymmetry of the jugular foramina. This can be useful when trying to decide if a small transverse sinus is due to thrombosis – a small sinus with a small jugular foramen is likely congenital.

Lumbar Spine Radiograph

16. Twelfth rib
17. Sacral promontory
18. Inferior articular facet of L5 vertebra
19. Spinous process of L3 vertebra
20. L2 nerve root

In the lumbar spine, the nerves exit beneath the pedicle of their respective vertebra. Vertically oriented superior and inferior articular facets give good vertebral stability such that vertebral malalignment should raise the possibility of a defect in the pars interarticularis, best seen on plain films in the oblique projection (Scotty dog view) or optimally demonstrated by CT.

Elbow Radiograph

21. Olecranon fossa left humerus
22. Normal anterior left humeral fat pad
23. Capitellum left humerus
24. Ossification centre of the olecranon of the left ulna
25. Ossification centre of the left medial epicondyle

The olecranon fossa may be fenestrated as a normal variant. The anterior fat pad is elevated in the presence of an elbow joint effusion but is less specific for fracture than an elevated posterior fat pad, which should never normally be visible.

MRI Head

26. Fourth ventricle
27. Nodule of cerebellum
28. Left posterior semicircular canal
29. Right vestibule
30. Left sixth cranial nerve

Barium Meal

31. Fundus of the stomach (barium in)
32. Antrum of the stomach
33. Second part of the duodenum
34. Duodenojejunal flexure
35. First part of the duodenum

Often, the primary purpose of the paediatric barium meal is to ascertain the position of the D-J flexure, in order to exclude malrotation. The D-J flexure should normally lie at the same level as the pylorus and lateral to the left pedicles.

Neonatal Cranial Ultrasound

36. Left caudate nucleus head
37. Corpus callosum
38. Falx cerebri
39. Left lateral ventricle
40. Right Sylvian fissure

Some degree of asymmetry of the lateral ventricles is usual. A cavum septum pellucidum is a usual feature in premature babies and often persists into infancy.

Shoulder Radiograph

41. Left proximal humeral growth plate
42. Coracoid process of left scapula
43. Left clavicle
44. Acromion of left scapula – ossification centre
45. Glenoid fossa of left scapula

The undulating growth plate of the proximal humerus is often mistaken for a fracture, as is the late to ossify secondary ossification centre of the acromion. Unossified acromion makes assessment of the acromioclavicular joint difficult in younger children.

Micturating Cystogram

46. Prostatic urethra
47. Membranous urethra
48. Bulbous urethra
49. Penile urethra
50. Unossified left triradiate cartilage

MRI Ankle

51. Achilles tendon
52. Calcaneum
53. Plantar fascia
54. Sesamoid bone at the first metatarsophalangeal joint
55. Sinus tarsi

CT Temporal Bone

56. Left incus
57. Left malleus
58. Apex of left petrous temporal bone
59. Left lambdoid suture
60. Left cochlear aperture

The incus is the cone and the malleus the ice cream. The cochlear aperture is the point of entry of the cochlear branch of the eighth cranial nerve into the cochlea. It may be small in congenital causes of sensorineural hearing loss.

MRI Pelvis

61. Left greater trochanter
62. Cauda equina
63. Right obturator internus
64. Urinary bladder
65. Left gluteus maximus

Chest Radiograph

66. Descending thoracic aorta
67. Stomach gas shadow
68. Lateral border right lobe of thymus
69. Ossification centre of left coracoid process of the scapula
70. Right horizontal (minor) fissure

The thymus is very variable in size and shape. It may be triangular when it abuts the horizontal fissure and often has a wavy outline. It never compresses or deviates other mediastinal structures, such as the trachea.

MRI Spine

71. Conus medullaris
72. Basivertebral vein of L3
73. Ligamentum flavum
74. Nucleus pulposus L4/5 intervertebral disc
75. Epidural fat

Intervertebral discs have a peripheral annulus fibrosus (dark on all MR sequences) and a central nucleus pulposus (intermediate signal). Normal basivertebral veins may enhance quite prominently following injection of gadolinium-based contrast material.

CT Chest

76. Main pulmonary artery
77. Calcified remnant of the ductus arteriosus
78. Azygous vein
79. Left pectoralis major
80. Carina

A fleck of calcification is often seen between the pulmonary artery and descending thoracic aorta at the site of the normally obliterated ductus arteriosus. It is less dense than a surgical ligation clip, which would also be at this site.

MRI Head

81. Right middle cerebral artery
82. Right cerebral peduncle
83. Aqueduct of Sylvius
84. Straight sinus
85. Crista galli

Ultrasound Hip

86. Right femoral head (unossified)
87. Right labrum
88. Right triradiate cartilage
89. Right ilium
90. Right acetabulum

This view is used to assess hip dysplasia. Alpha and beta angles as well as subjective morphological assessment of the acetabulum along with dynamic manoeuvres can be used to quantify the degree of developmental hip dysplasia.

MRI Knee

91. Patella (unossified cartialage)
92. Distal femoral epiphysis
93. Posterior cruciate ligament
94. Quadriceps tendon
95. Gastrocnemius

Ultrasound Abdomen

96. Aorta
97. Pyloric canal
98. Head of pancreas
99. Left lobe of liver
100. Right rectus abdominus

Hypertrophic pyloric stenosis is suggested in the presence of a thickened, elongated pylorus (single muscle thickness >3 mm, canal length >17 mm). This may be associated with prominent gastric peristaltic waves and a failure to see opening of the pyloric canal after a test feed.

Test 10: Normal Anatomical Variants

10

P. Borg et al., *Radiological Anatomy for FRCR Part 1*,
DOI 10.1007/978-3-642-41166-3_10, © Springer-Verlag Berlin Heidelberg 2014

CT Abdomen

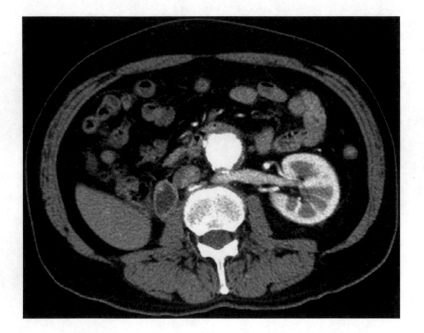

Question 1

Name the normal variant

CT Head

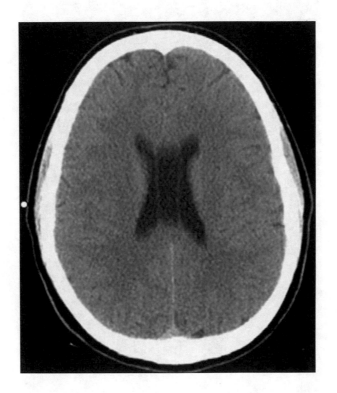

Question 2

Name the normal variant

Abdominal Radiograph

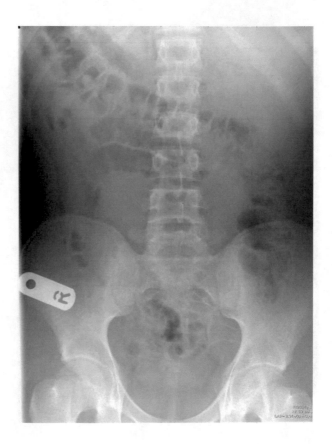

Question 3a

Name the normal variant

(Continued): Chest Radiograph

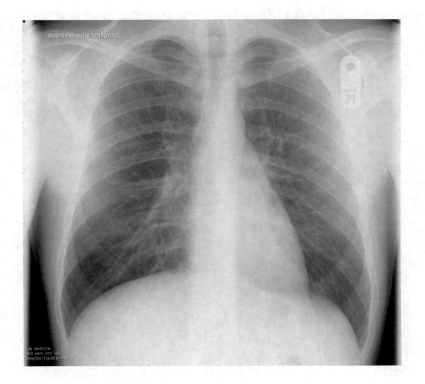

Question 3b

Name the normal variant

CT Abdomen

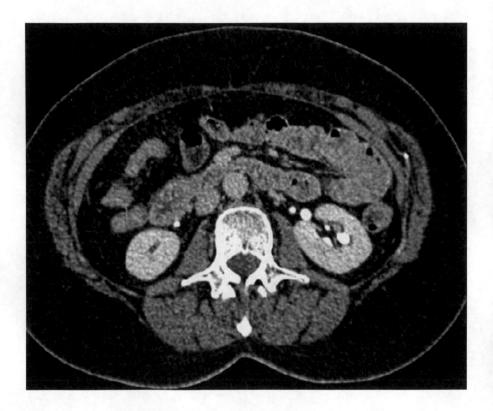

Question 4

Name the normal variant

Foot Radiograph

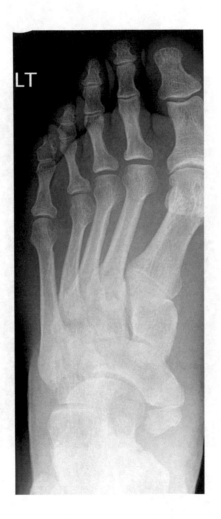

Question 5

Name the normal variant

Shoulder Radiograph

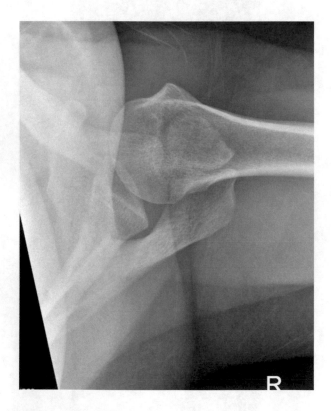

Question 6

Name the normal variant

Chest Radiograph

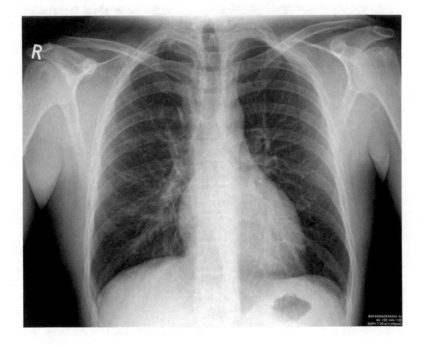

Question 7

Name the normal variant

Chest Radiograph

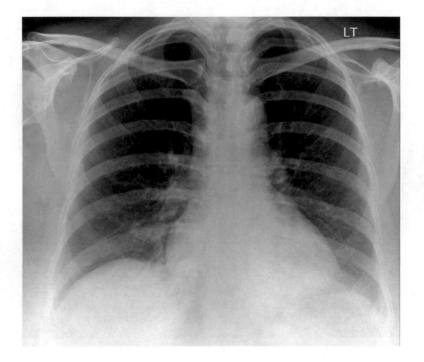

Question 8

Name the normal variant

CT Abdomen

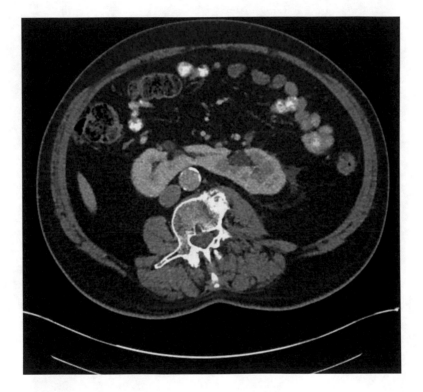

Question 9

Name the normal variant

Hand Radiograph

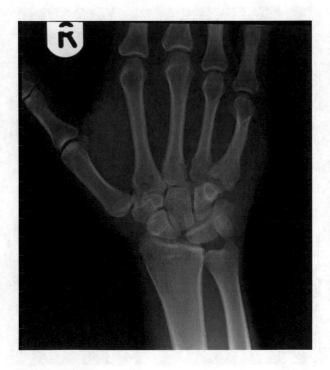

Question 10

Name the normal variant

Foot Radiograph

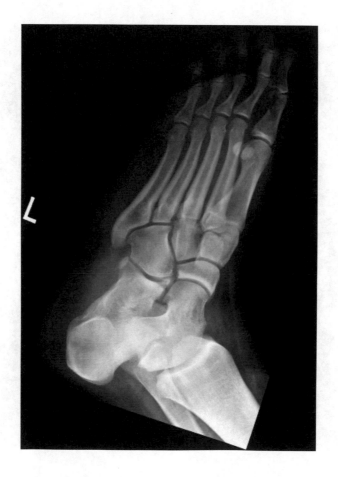

Question 11

Name the normal variant

CT Abdomen

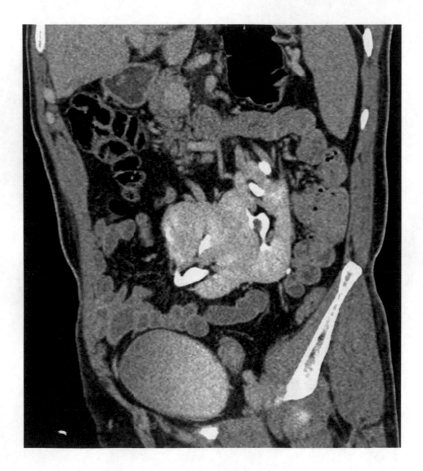

(Continued): CT Abdomen (3D Reconstruction)

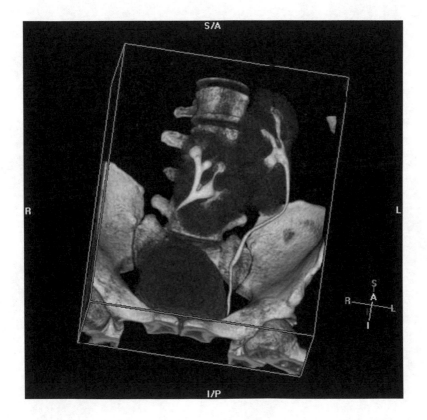

Question 12b

Name the normal variant

CT Chest

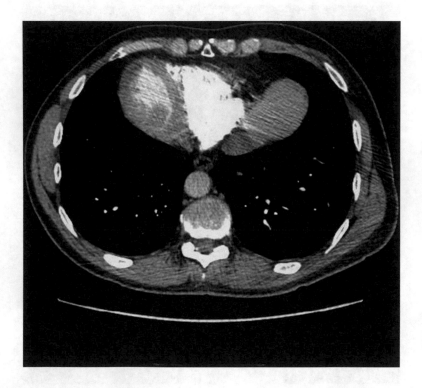

Question 13

Name the normal variant

Chest Radiograph

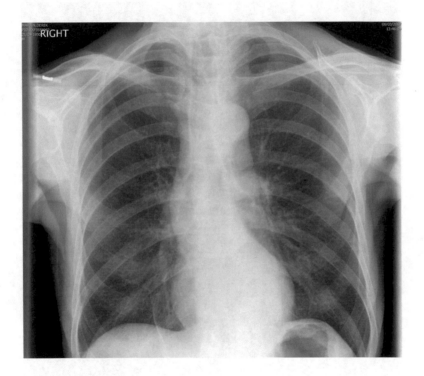

Question 14

Name the normal variant

MRCP

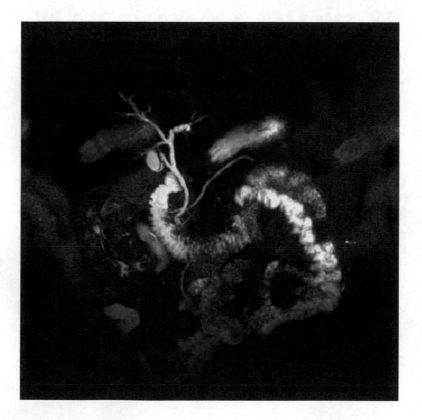

CT Chest

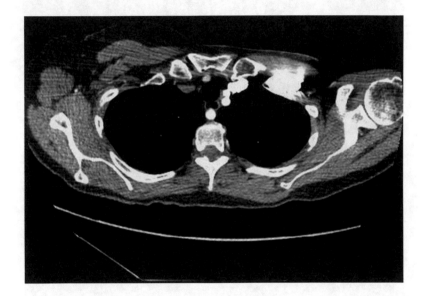

Question 16

Name the normal variant

Chest Radiograph

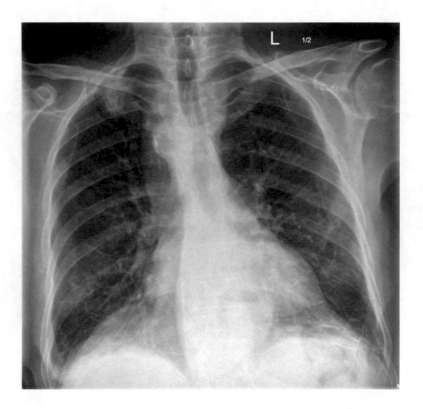

Question 17

Name the normal variant

Coronal CT Abdomen

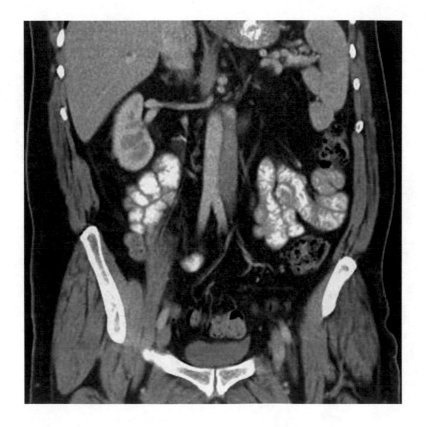

Question 18a

Name the normal variant

(Axial) CT Abdomen

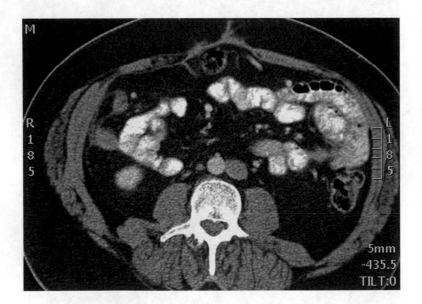

Question 18b

Name the normal variant

Barium Meal

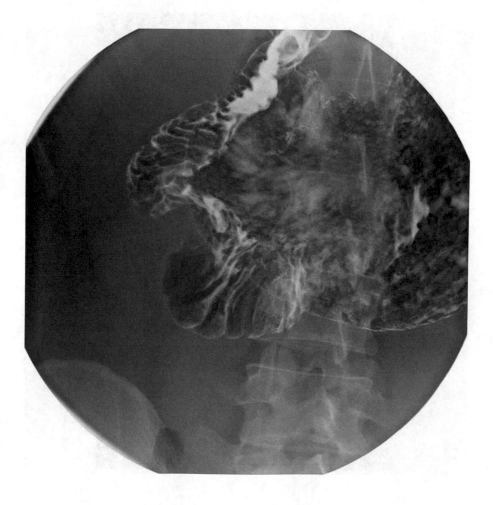

Ankle Radiograph

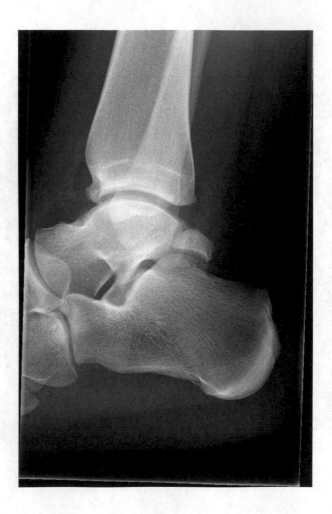

Question 20

Name the normal variant

Test 10: Normal Anatomical Variants Answers

CT Abdomen

Retroaortic left renal vein
Retroaortic left renal vein occurs as part of the complex development of the inferior vena cava. The exact incidence is unknown (estimated 3 %), but it is increasingly being reported with high resolution images on CT and MRI.

Patients are usually asymptomatic, but compression of the left renal vein may cause haematuria, flank pain and varicoceles. It is important to report a retroaortic left renal vein if a patient is going to have a nephrectomy, either for malignancy or as a living kidney donor.

CT Head

Cavum vergae
A cavum septum pellucidum separates the frontal horns of the lateral ventricles, anterior to the foramina of Monro. A cavum vergae cannot exist without a cavum septum pellucidum but extends posterior to the splenium of the corpus callosum.

Abdominal Radiograph

Complete situs inversus
Abdominal situs refers to the position of the liver and stomach. On this abdominal X-ray the liver is seen on the left side of the abdomen as is the caecum, and gas within the stomach can be seen on the right. This is seen in complete situs inversus. Remember to look at the side marker to ensure that this diagnosis is correct.

Situs ambiguous is when the liver is symmetrical, and the stomach is seen in the midline.

(Continued): Chest Radiograph

Situs inversus (same patient's CXR)
Thoracic situs refers to the position of the tracheobronchial tree. In situs inversus the right main bronchus is longer than the left main bronchus, the left upper lobe bronchus is superior to the left pulmonary artery, and the right upper lobe bronchus is inferior to the right pulmonary artery. It is associated with dextrocardia, as in this example. The stomach bubble can be seen below the right hemidiaphragm.

Beware of the side marker – in this example the image has been deliberately shown to make you look at the side marker and spot the abnormality.

CT Abdomen

Duplex left kidney
Duplex kidney is seen in 4 % population. It is in the most common normal variant in the urinary tract. On ultrasound, a band of tissue is seen to separate the two moieties, and if there is distension of the kidney, two ureters may be visualised.

Foot Radiograph

Os tibiale externum
Sesamoid bones are relatively common on foot radiographs. Os tibiale externum is seen medial to the tuberosity of the navicular within the tendon of the tibialis posterior muscle.

Shoulder Radiograph

Os acromiale
This relatively common accessory ossicle results from failure of fusion of the secondary ossification centre of the acromion. Not to be mistaken for a fracture!

Chest Radiograph

Azygous fissure
The azygous fissure is seen due to the azygous vein passing through the apical portion of the right upper lobe. The fissure contains four layers of pleura (two parietal and two visceral) which is why the fissure is more prominent than the reminder of the fissures. It is present in 1 % of postmortem specimens but only seen on 0.4 % CXR.

Chest Radiograph

Left cervical rib
A cervical rib is a normal variant but can cause clinical symptoms. Patients may present with tingling and numbness of the hand. A cervical rib is a bony or fibrous band between C7 and the first rib. They are seen in 1–2 % people. Fifty percent are bilateral, but they are often asymmetrical.

CT Abdomen

Horseshoe kidney
Kidneys may fuse during development leading to a horseshoe kidney. This is seen in 1 in 700 births and is the most common fusion anomaly. The kidney is fused

across the midline. The isthmus, joining the kidneys, may be composed of functioning renal tissue or just fibrous tissue. A horseshoe kidney is more prone to injury than usual as it lies across the vertebral column.

The axis of the kidneys is abnormal, with the lower pole more medial than the upper pole. The isthmus lies anterior to the aorta and IVC but behind the IMA.

Hand Radiograph

Coalition of lunate and triquetral
Carpal coalition is relatively uncommon but is a recognised normal variant. Look at the carpal bones, identify each one on an image, and you should be able to notice coalition when present.

Foot Radiograph

Os vesalianum fused to base of 5th metatarsal.
Within the foot, there can be multiple sesamoid bones, which you will not be expected to name. This image shows an example of where one of these, the os vesalianum, has fused to the fifth metatarsal. This may cause patient symptoms and is important to pick up.

CT Abdomen

Crossed fused renal ectopia
The lower kidney is usually the one that is ectopic. Abnormal rotation is present, and renal pelvises may face opposite directions. This is seen in 1/1,000 births, and the incidence of associated anomalies is low. There is a slightly increased incidence of renal calculi.

CT Chest

Dextrocardia
On this CT image, the cardiac chambers are in an abnormal position, and the heart is on the right side of the thorax.

Chest Radiograph

Inferior accessory fissure
Inferior accessory fissure is seen in 8 % CXR and 20 % HRCT. It separates the medial basal segment from the other right lower lobe segments. It is also known as Twinings' line. It is found on 30–50 % postmortem specimens.

MRCP

Pancreas divisum
Failure of fusion of the dorsal and ventral moieties of the pancreas results in the anterosuperior part of the head and the body and tail draining via the accessory papilla, with the posteroinferior part of the head draining to the ampulla.

CT Chest

Aberrant right subclavian artery
This variant is seen in 0.5 %. The right subclavian artery arises distal to the left subclavian artery and passes to the right, posterior to the oesophagus. In the example given, an artery can be seen behind the oesophagus, where no vessel is usually seen.

Chest Radiograph

Right-sided aortic arch
Seen in 1–2 % of people due to persistence of the right aortic arch and right descending aorta and regression of the left aortic arch. The arch courses to the right of the trachea and oesophagus, over the right main bronchus. It crosses over the lower thoracic spine and passes through the left hemidiaphragm. It is often associated with other vascular and cardiac anomalies.

CT Abdomen

Left-sided inferior vena cava
Seen in 0.2–0.5 % people due to persistence of the left and regression of the right supracardinal vein. The left IVC usually joins the left renal vein.

Barium Meal

Annular pancreas
This results from abnormal migration of the ventral pancreatic bud. The pancreas surrounds and can cause obstruction of the duodenum. It appears as an annular constriction of the second part of the duodenum on barium studies. There is an increased incidence of pancreatitis and peptic ulcer disease.

On CT, soft tissue arising from the pancreas can be seen surrounding the duodenum. On the barium study, there is a smooth circumferential narrowing of the duodenum, and using the two studies in conjunction, a definite diagnosis of annular pancreas can be made.

Ankle Radiograph

Os trigonum
Seen in 7 % of people, it can sometimes be mistaken for a fracture. It may be a source of pain and is therefore important to recognise and report on.

Printed in the United States
By Bookmasters